New Drugs on the Street: Changing Inner City Patterns of Illicit Consumption

New Drugs on the Street: Changing Inner City Patterns of Illicit Consumption has been co-published simultaneously as *Journal of Ethnicity in Substance Abuse*, Volume 4, Number 2 2005.

The *Journal of Ethnicity in Substance Abuse*™ is the successor title to *Drugs & Society,* which changed title after Vol. 16, No. 1/2 2000. The journal is renumbered to start as Vol. 1, No. 1 2002.

New Drugs on the Street: Changing Inner City Patterns of Illicit Consumption, edited by Merrill Singer, PhD (Vol. 4, No. 2, 2005). *"ESSENTIAL READING for anyone in the drug use area who wants to be brought up-to-date on the current state of the field. This edited work provides an excellent look at a number of emerging drug use trends. This includes new drugs appearing in particular areas, drugs appearing among different subpopulations, and gaining a better understanding of the composition of drugs already being used." (Scott Clair, PhD, Associate Scientist, Partnerships in Prevention Science Institute, Iowa State University)*

New Drugs on the Street: Changing Inner City Patterns of Illicit Consumption

Merrill Singer, PhD
Editor

New Drugs on the Street: Changing Inner City Patterns of Illicit Consumption has been co-published simultaneously as *Journal of Ethnicity in Substance Abuse*, Volume 4, Number 2 2005.

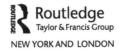

Routledge
Taylor & Francis Group

NEW YORK AND LONDON

First Published by

The Haworth Press, Inc., 10 Alice Street, Binghamton, NY 13904-1580 USA

Transferred to Digital Printing 2011 by Routladge
711 Third Avenue, New York, NY 10017
2 Park Square, Milton Park, Abingdon, Oxon, OX14 4RN

New Drugs on the Street: Changing Inner City Patterns of Illicit Consumption has been co-published simultaneously as *Journal of Ethnicity in Substance Abuse*™, Volume 4, Number 2 2005.

Cover design by Marylouise Doyle
Cover illustration by Jacob Singer

Library of Congress Cataloging-in-Publication Data

New drugs on the street: changing inner city patterns of illicit consumption/Merrill Singer.
    p. cm.
    "Co-published simultaneously as Journal of Ethnicity in Substance Abuse, Volume 4, Number 2, 2005."
    Includes bibliographical references and index.
    ISBN-10: 0-7890-3050-0 (hard cover : alk. paper)
    ISBN-10: 0-7890-3051-9 (soft cover : alk. paper)
    ISBN-13: 978-0-7890-3050-4 (hard cover: alk.paper)
    ISBN-13: 978-0-7890-3051-1 (soft cover: alk.paper)
1. Drug abuse–United States. 2. Substance abuse–United States. 3. Drugs of abuse–United States. 4. Urban Youth–Drug use–United States. 5. Minorities–Drug use–United States. 6. Inner cities–United States. I. Singer, Merrill. II. Journal of Ethnicity in Substance Abuse.

HV5825.N428 2005
362.29'09173'2–dc22
                                                        2005013434

New Drugs on the Street: Changing Inner City Patterns of Illicit Consumption

CONTENTS

ABOUT THE EDITOR

Merrill Singer, PhD, is Associate Director of the Hispanic Health Council (HHC) and Director of the HHC's Center for Community Health Research in Hartford, CT. He has been with the HHC for 23 years and has helped to lead the organization into national prominence as a community-based minority health research institute. Dr. Singer has been the Principal Investigator on a continuous series of federal and foundation funded drinking, drug use, and AIDS prevention grants since 1984, and currently is the Principal Investigator on three studies. He has published over 130 articles and writes a regular column for the Society for Applied Anthropology Newsletter and is author, co-author, or co-editor of ten books. He is past Associate Editor of the *Journal of Medical Anthropology*, is the current Book Editor of *Medical Anthropology Quarterly*, and is an editorial board member of the *Journal of Ethnicity in Substance Abuse* and *The International Journal of Drug Policy*. Dr. Singer was selected as the first recipient of the new Practicing Anthropology Award by the Society for Medical Anthropology.

New Drugs on the Street:
An Introduction

Merrill Singer, PhD

One crisp morning in the spring of 1999, Marvin Byrd, a resident of the Asylum Hill neighborhood of Hartford, took a meandering walk down a busy city street bereft of shoes or socks. The 60s, and their naturalist acceptance of shoelessness, were long past. More so, walking barefoot on litter-strewn streets was risky business. His neighbors, consequently, thought Byrd had gone crazy. But his curious behavior, which caught the expansive attention of a newspaper reporter covering drug abuse in the city (Comer, 2000), was not a unique event. As explained by a participant in a Hispanic Health Council study of changing patterns of illicit drug consumption:

> That is why you be . . . you don't feel the cold, you just be warm walking around with no jacket. You feel light, like you're walking on the air.

The drug that causes this strange effect on users, a prepared mixture of several different illicit and legal substances that is sold under a variety of street names, including "dust," "illy," "hemmy," "wet," and "tical," is one of the *new drugs of the street.*

Over the last decade, researchers, treatment providers, and drug users themselves have witnessed the introduction and street use of a steady

[Haworth co-indexing entry note]: "New Drugs on the Street: An Introduction." Singer, Merrill. Co-published simultaneously in *Journal of Ethnicity in Substance Abuse* (The Haworth Press, Inc.) Vol. 4, No. 2, 2005, pp. 1-7; and: *New Drugs on the Street: Changing Inner City Patterns of Illicit Consumption* (ed: Merrill Singer) The Haworth Press, Inc., 2005, pp. 1-7. Single or multiple copies of this article are available for a fee from The Haworth Document Delivery Service [1-800-HAWORTH, 9:00 a.m. - 5:00 p.m. (EST). E-mail address: docdelivery@haworthpress.com].

Available online at http://www.haworthpress.com/web/JESA
doi:10.1300/J233v04n02_01

1

stream of new (or renewed) psychotropic drugs. During this period, the term "street drug user" has become a standard term in the drug literature. Referring primarily to inner city substance users who are forced by poverty, discrimination, and their addiction into a far more visible and public pattern of drug acquisition and consumption than their wealthier, suburban or more rural drug using counterparts (Singer and Easton, 2004), the term draws attention to the context of drug use as a central issue of social and public health concern. While it may take place in abandoned buildings, dark alleyways, isolated sections of cemeteries, recessed doorways, wooded parks, discarded cars, or similar somewhat shielded locations, street drug use attracts most of the attention that the media, the police, and the War on Drugs more broadly devote to the consumer-side of the drug problem in American society.

Commonly, the U.S. "drug problem" is viewed as the illicit consumption of substances like cocaine and heroin and, to a lesser degree, marijuana. Importantly, however, the street drug use scene is not stagnant; instead it has undergone rapid changes in recent years as new drugs, old drugs in new forms, alternative ways of using existing drugs, and fresh populations of drug users have entered the scene. This collection of papers is concerned with exploring these changes, with special concern for shifting patterns of drug use among U.S. urban populations of African and Hispanic origin.

The new drugs of the street, including substances like ecstasy, dust, illicit benzodiazepines and narcotic analgesics, flavored cigars, and high-THC marijuana, thus far have not transformed street drug use, in that older patterns remain dominant even as important new trends become evident. Heroin injection, for example, has had a primary place in street drug use repertoires since the late 1940s and early 1950s. For inner city youth during the post-War War II period, however–an era during which earlier street drug use practices had been disrupted by the war–heroin was a new drug on the street. The appearance of heroin and its impact on inner city communities after the Second World War–a period during which drug research was all but non-existent–is well-described in a number of autobiographies of individuals who became street drug users at the time (Singer, 1999). One such account, by jazz musician Art Pepper (1994:86), who first used heroin in 1950, summarizes the immediate impact of the drug on his life in words that apply as well to many new street drug users at the time:

> All I can say is, at the moment I saw that I'd found peace of mind. Synthetically produced, but after what I'd been through and all the

things I'd done, to trade that misery for total happiness–that was it, you know, that was it. I realized it. I realized that from that moment on I would be, if you want to use the word, a junkie. That's the word they used. That's the word they still use. That is what I became at that moment. That's what I practiced; and that's what I still am. And that's what I will die as–a junkie.

As he had foreseen, on June 15, 1982, Pepper died in a California hospital, still a junkie. Over twenty years later, heroin remains in common street use, although heightened levels of drug purity and fear of AIDS have contributed to changing use patterns and new populations of users (Neaigus, 1998).

In the late 1980s and early 1990s, cocaine became a new drug of the city. Powder cocaine, of course, was not a new drug at the time; it had been in use in American cities since early in the country's history (Singer, 2005). During the 1980s, cocaine use even passed through a chic phase, becoming the expensive and fashionable drug of choice from A-list Hollywood parties to plush-carpeted New York office suites. As some of the harsher realities of sustained cocaine use began to curb its appeal among society's trendsetters, however, a new version of the drug was invented and marketed by illicit suppliers. By "cooking" cocaine powder with a little water and sodium bicarbonate, dealers found they could produce a rock version of the drug–called crack, probably because of the popping and snapping sound made as the drug was being made–that could be profitably sold for as little as $5 per rapid high-producing piece, making it viable for street-level distribution in the inner city (including to suburbanites who use the inner city as a drive-in/drive-out drug mall). The effect of the renewed form of cocaine on the street drug scene has been widely documented by researchers, with special reference to new populations of street drug users such as women, as well as to the common role of crack in street violence (Inciardi, Lockwood and Pottieger, 1993; Ratner, 1993; Sterk, 1999).

During the first two decades of the AIDS epidemic–the 1980s and 1990s–heroin, powder cocaine, and crack were the primary street drugs garnering research attention. Speedball, a combination of cocaine and heroin, was one of the few drugs on the street that became a new topic of street drug research. Other drug combinations, polydrug use generally, and the mixing of sex and drug use also emerged as issues of concern (Booth, Watters and Chitwood, 1993). Later the re-conversion of crack into an injectable liquid form (through mixture with vinegar or citric acid) caught on and became a lesser known but still not uncommon new street drug use practice (Carlson, Falck and Siegal, 2000; Hunter, Donoghoe and Stimson, 1995). In the West–although not for a number of years in other parts of the country–the spread of methamphetamine (Gorman, Morgan and Lambert, 1995; Urbina and Jones, 2004) was also recognized as a dangerous new threat to the health of street drug users. Finally, new street drug use locations, especially shooting galleries and crack houses (sites with varying local names such as "get offs"), became topics of research interest (Bourgois, 1998; Des Jarlais, Friedman and Strug, 1986; Golub and Johnson, 1996; Ouellet et al., 1991; Page, Smith and Kane, 1991). Until the end of the 1990s, these had been the drug use practices, contexts, and populations that largely had defined the street drug scene (Kral et al., 1998), although it was recognized that marijuana and alcohol (although less studied in this context) were consumed regularly and often in large quantities by street heroin and cocaine users.

With the transition to the 21st century, however, a new wave of drug use with its own evolving set of dynamics began to unfold. One source of change was the late night dance club, a recreational site that pulled together diverse populations and created an arena for learning about, gaining access to, and experimenting with, drugs used by other populations. As seen in the papers by Eiserman and Schensul and their respective co-authors in this collection, the clubs became a nexus between the inner city and suburbia, with population and drug mixing leading to the movement of drugs like ecstasy beyond the dance scene to street consumption. Thus far, other club drugs, like ketamine or GHB, while they have some limited street use, have not become new drugs of the street. Indeed, unlike ecstasy, many street drug users have never heard of, let alone tried them. Even ecstasy is a relative expensive drug for street drug users, and while it has found a market on the street, as well as a place in hip hop music and other popular urban cultural expressions, its use is far from universal among street drug users.

A lengthy list of tranquilizer and pain-relieving drugs that Vivian and co-authors in this set of papers refer to as "under the counter pharmaceuticals" because they have been diverted from prescription-controlled to illicit non-medical consumption, also have rapidly diffused to the inner city in recent years. In some places, pharmaceutical narcotics are now outstripping heroin in street sales and use. On the street, drug appeal is defined by effect, availability, and price. Street drug users often report that they like pharmaceuticals because their content is consistent and effects predictable, they are readily and widely available, and they are affordable as individual pills even for generally impoverished street drug users.

The use of dust, which is examined by Singer and colleagues in this set of papers, reflects two patterns of the new street drug scene: drug mixing and the renewal of drugs that had been in use earlier on the street but had subsequently declined in popularity. Dust is a mixture of several substances and, because of decentralized local production, content no doubt is inconsistent. Commonly, dust contains phencyclidine (PCP), which was first produced (and later largely discarded) as a pharmaceutical anesthetic. Other ingredients can include embalming fluid and marijuana. The reappearance of PCP is somewhat surprising given the negative attitudes about its effects that developed during its last wave of use in the 1960s-1970s. While, as the opening paragraphs above suggest, negative effects continue to be reported, one purpose of mixing it with other substances may be to limit the intensity of undesired behavioral and experiential outcomes. Conversely, as Holland et al. (1998) have argued, they may be but window dressing designed to market an old and out-of-favor drug by wrapping it in exotic new chemical packaging.

As indicated above, study of the new drugs of the street entails as well an examination of new drug users and even new drug sellers (as the latter change also can have effect on drug content). An unfortunate aspect of contemporary drug use is that during the era of AIDS many new populations have begun using drugs including adopting the most risky forms of drug consumption, such as direct syringe sharing. The final paper in this collection examines one such population: Haitian youth and young adults. While drug use in Haiti, beyond marijuana and alcohol, was minimal, among individuals who have migrated (or fled) from that troubled island to southern Florida, drug use and distribution are beginning to take hold. This finding may (or in the future may) be the case as well for other foreign-born populations that have migrated to U.S. cities in large numbers in recent years, such as Bosnians, Brazilians, and Sudanese and other African refugees.

Drugs have taken a significant toll on city populations, more so since the rise of the AIDS epidemic. Prevention and treatment programs have never kept pace with the scale of the problem, resulting in it being far easier to get drugs than drug treatment in the U.S. (Singer, 2004). Moreover, to be effective such programs must stay abreast of the new drugs on the street (including their use patterns, effects, and populations and contexts of use), and be guided by a recognition of drug use as a dynamic process that is sensitive to other changes in society, including the uneven impact of the War on Drugs (which may reduce the availability of one drug only to increase the availability of another), the profit-driven strategies of drug suppliers (who, like licit entrepreneurs, are ever on the lookout for new markets and marketing devices), the globalization of the economy (which facilitates the flow of goods, jobs, and populations across national boundaries), the spread of multi-disease syndemics (such as the intertwinement of drug abuse, violence, AIDS and other blood-borne diseases), structural patterns of discrimination and marginalization (that contribute to illicit self-medication of distress and social suffering), and unhealthy health policies (like the federal ban on funding for syringe exchange). In light of this set of factors that facilitate and may help to speed-up rates of social change, the purpose of this set of papers is to draw attention to the importance of paying ever closer attention to the drugs on the street as they undergo new waves of change in the new century.

REFERENCES

Booth, R., J. Watters, and D. Chitwood (1993) HIV Risk-related sex behaviors among injection drug users, crack smokers, and injection drug users who smoke crack. *American Journal of Public Health* 83 (8): 1144-1148.

Bourgois, P. (1998) Just another night in a shooting gallery. *Theory, Culture and Society* 15 (2): 37-66.

Carlson, R., R. Falck, and H. Siegal (2000) Crack cocaine injection in the Heartland: An ethnographic perspective. *Medical Anthropology* 18 (4): 305-323.

Comer, A. (2000) The wildness of wet. *Hartford Courant* March 26, p. 3.

Des Jarlais, D., S. Friedman, and D. Strug (1986) AIDS and needle sharing within the IV-drug use subculture. In *The Social Dimensions of AIDS*. Douglas Feldman and Thomas Johnson (eds.), pp. 111-125. New York: Praeger.

Golub, A. and B. Johnson (1996) The crack epidemic: Empirical findings support an hypothesized diffusion of innovation process. *Socioeconomic Planning Science* 30: 221-231.

Gorman, E. M., P. Morgan, and E. Lambert (1995) Qualitative research considerations and other issues in the study of Methamphetamine use among men who have sex with other men. In *Qualitative Methods in Drug Abuse and HIV Research*. E. Lambert, R. Ashery, and R. Needle (eds.), pp. 156-181. *NIDA Research Monograph* 157. Rockville, MD: National Institute on Drug Abuse.

Holland, J., L. Nelson, P. Ravikumar, and E. William (1998) Embalming fluid-soaked Marijuana: New high or new guise for PCP? *Journal of Psychoactive Drugs* 30 (2): 215-219.

Hunter, G., M. Donoghoe, and G. Stimson (1995) Crack use and injection on the increase among injection drug users in London. *Addiction* 90: 1397-1400.

Inciardi, J., D. Lockwood and A. Pottieger (1993) *Women and Crack-Cocaine*. New York: Macmillan Publishing Co.

Kral, A., R. Bluthenthal, R. Booth, and J. Watters (1998 HIV seroprevalence among street-recruited injection drug and crack cocaine users in 16 U.S. municipalities. *American Journal of Public Health* 88 (1): 108-111.

Neaigus, A. (1998) Trends in the noninjected use of Heroin and factors associated with the transition to injection. In *Heroin in the Age of Crack Cocaine*. J. Inciardi and L. Harrison (Eds.), pp. 131-159. Thousand Oaks: Sage Publications, Inc.

Ouellet, L., A. Jimenez, W. Johnson, and W. Wiebel (1991) Shooting galleries and HIV disease: Variations in places for injecting drugs. *Crime and Delinquency* 37 (1): 64-85.

Page, J. B., P. Smith, and N. Kane (1991) Shooting galleries, their proprietors and implications for prevention. *Drugs & Society* 5 (1/2): 69-85.

Pepper, A. and L. Pepper (1994) *Straight Life: The Story of Art Pepper*. New York: Da Capo Press.

Ratner, M. (1993) Sex, drugs, and public policy: Studying and understanding the sex-for-crack phenomenon. In *Crack Pipe as Pimp: An Ethnographic Investigation of Sex-for-Crack Exchanges*. M. Ratner (Ed.), pp. 1-36. New York: Lexington Books.

Singer, M. (1999) The ethnography of street drug use before AIDS: A historic review. In *Cultural, Observational, and Epidemiological Approaches in the Prevention of Drug Abuse and HIV/AIDS*. P. Marshall, M. Singer, and M. Clatts (Eds.), pp. 228-264. Bethesda, MD: National Institute on Drug Abuse.

Singer, M. (2004) Why it is easier to get drugs than drug treatment? In *Unhealthy Health Policy: A Critical Anthropological Examination*. A. Castro and M. Singer (Eds.). Walnut Creek, CA: Altamira Press.

Singer, M. (2005) *Something Dangerous: Emergent and Changing Illicit Drug Use and Community Health*. Prospect Heights, IL: Waveland Press.

Singer, M. and D. Easton (in press) Ethnographic research on drugs and HIV/AIDS in ethnocultural communities. In *The Handbook of Ethical Research with Ethnocultural Populations and Communities*. C. Fisher and J. Trimble (Eds.). Sage Publications.

Sterk, C. (1999) *Fast Lives: Women Who Use Crack Cocaine*. Philadelphia: Temple University Press.

Urbina, A. and K. Jones (2004) Crystal Methamphetamine, its analogues, and HIV infection: Medical and psychiatric aspects of a new epidemic. *Clinical and Infectious Diseases* 38 (6): 890-4.

"Rollin' on E":
A Qualitative Analysis of Ecstasy Use Among Inner City Adolescents and Young Adults

Julie M. Eiserman, MA
Sarah Diamond, PhD
Jean J. Schensul, PhD

SUMMARY. Ecstasy use has spread beyond the rave and club scenes into other arenas of party culture, and from middle-class America to working-class and low-income neighborhoods of large cities. In order to explore ecstasy use among inner city adolescents and young adults, we

Julie M. Eiserman is Associate Research Scientist at the Hispanic Health Council. Sarah Diamond is a Research Associate at the Institute for Community Research. Jean J. Schensul is Senior Scientist and Founding Director of the Institute for Community Research.

Address correspondence to: Julie M. Eiserman, Hispanic Health Council, 175 Main Street, Hartford, CT 06106 (E-mail: juliee@hispanichealth.com).

The authors express appreciation for the support provided for this paper from other Pathways' team members: Merrill Singer, PhD; Margaret Weeks, PhD; Raul Pino, MD; Lori Broomhall, PhD; Cristina Huebner, MA; Scott Clair, PhD; Gary Burkholder, PhD; Mark Convey, MA; Jose Garcia, MA; Gustavo Lopez, BA; and Rey Bermudez, BA.

Research for this paper was supported by NIDA Grant # R01-DA-11421 and OAR Supplement # DA-11421-02S1.

[Haworth co-indexing entry note]: "'Rollin' on E': A Qualitative Analysis of Ecstasy Use Among Inner City Adolescents and Young Adults." Eiserman, Julie M., Sarah Diamond, and Jean J. Schensul. Co-published simultaneously in *Journal of Ethnicity in Substance Abuse* (The Haworth Press, Inc.) Vol. 4, No. 2, 2005, pp. 9-38; and: *New Drugs on the Street: Changing Inner City Patterns of Illicit Consumption* (ed: Merrill Singer) The Haworth Press, Inc., 2005, pp. 9-38. Single or multiple copies of this article are available for a fee from The Haworth Document Delivery Service [1-800-HAWORTH, 9:00 a.m. - 5:00 p.m. (EST). E-mail address: docdelivery@haworthpress.com].

conducted in-depth interviews with 23 poly-drug users who had used ecstasy, in Hartford, CT. Most users reported positive experiences while on the drug. Negative experiences were most often related to poly-drug mixing. However, heavy users (40+ times ever used) experienced negative aftereffects, which led them to decide to decrease or halt their use. Some participants discussed using ecstasy during sex, and irregular use of condoms. These findings point to the need for more in-depth research on MDMA use within inner city settings, with a particular focus on ethnic and cultural context, self-controlled drug use, poly-drug mixing, and sex risk behaviors. *[Article copies available for a fee from The Haworth Document Delivery Service: 1-800-HAWORTH. E-mail address: <docdelivery@ haworthpress.com> Website: <http://www.HaworthPress.com> © 2005 by The Haworth Press, Inc. All rights reserved.]*

KEYWORDS. Ecstasy, inner city, young adults, adolescents, drug use, risk

INTRODUCTION

Ecstasy (MDMA, or 3,4-Methylenedioxymethamphetamine) was developed and marketed in the mid-1970s as a therapeutic drug, useful because of its capacity to induce empathy and social attachment. In 1985, it became a controlled substance in the U.S. In spite of that, by the mid-1990s, ecstasy or "E" had been integrated into the rave youth culture in Europe, Australia, and the large urban centers of the United States (Hitzler, 2002; Lenton, Boys, and Norcross, 1997; Yacoubian, Boyle, Harding, and Loftus, 2003). The use of ecstasy in the United States reached its peak in 2001 (Johnston, O'Malley, and Bachman, 2003). In response to fears of a growing ecstasy epidemic, the government began increasing sentencing guidelines and mounting national campaigns to warn the public of the hazards of using ecstasy. The Illicit Drug Anti-Proliferation Act of 2003 (S.226), formerly known as the "Rave Act," penalized rave organizers, club owners, and entertainment promoters for the manufacture, sale, and use of drugs at their events. Due to these concerted government efforts, ecstasy use has fallen in the past few years. However, ecstasy continues to be widely used and is spreading to new users (Singer, in press). Furthermore, ecstasy use has spread beyond the rave and club scenes into other arenas of party culture, and from the suburbs and middle-class America to working-class and low-income neighborhoods of large cities (Schensul et al., this issue).

The continued use of ecstasy among adolescents and young adults seems to be related to the properties of the drug, which are uniquely suited to modern-day youth culture. Its stimulant properties make MDMA useful for enduring long periods of dancing and all-night activities. MDMA also enhances physical sensation and induces an immediate sense of intimacy and connectedness between people with no prior association (Hinchliff, 2001; Reynolds, 1999). Thus, the drug is appealing to adolescents and young adults who feel ill at ease in social settings; who wish to make new friends or acquaintances; or who are seeking new sexual partners and experiences. Moreover, ecstasy users view the drug as having broad-based "benefit" and being low "risk" (Parker, Aldridge, and Measham, 1998). However, government officials and the medical community see ecstasy use as a significant public health problem, due to research demonstrating both short-term and long-term health risks. Ecstasy use has been linked to hyperthermia, depression, and impaired cognitive functioning (Haddad, Strickland, Anderson, Deakin, and Dursun, 2002; Parrott et al., 2002; Parrott, Sisk, and Turner, 2000; Rodgers, 2000).

Most of the scientific literature on ecstasy focuses on the epidemiology of ecstasy use, especially on prevalence in high-risk populations (e.g., rave and gay circuit party attendees), or on the negative dimensions of short-term and long-term consequences (Agar and Reisinger, 2004; Arria, Yacoubian, Fost, and Wish, 2002; Gross, Barrett, Shestowsky, and Pihl, 2002; Klitzman, Pope, and Hudson, 2000; Lee, Galanter, Dermatis, and McDowell, 2003; Mansergh et al., 2001; Ross, Mattison, and Franklin, 2003). National drug awareness campaigns have depicted ecstasy, along with other so-called designer or club drugs, as a risky dangerous drug which leads to dehydration, depression, and even death (sometimes referred to as ecstasy's three D's). Popular entertainment media portray ecstasy as a fashionable drug, linked with alcohol use and an expensive lifestyle. Hip hop music has endorsed it as a drug that enhances sexual experience, but may have negative consequences (Diamond, Bermudez, and Schensul, under review). As McElrath has noted, mass media messages about ecstasy are mediated by the perceptions and experiences of adolescents and young adults themselves (McElrath and McEvoy, 2001). These personal experiences are not only shared in social networks, but they are also conveyed in a variety of popular locations on the Internet which provide online bulletin boards for users to share their drug experiences, e.g., Erowid.org, DanceSafe.org, etc. (Brewer, 2003; Falck, Carlson, Wang, and Siegal, 2004). These interactive Internet sites tend to take a neutral stance toward drug use and a positive stance toward drug users and harm reduction.

The research on socialization into ecstasy use, the effects of ecstasy on sensation and behavior including qualitative descriptions of the range of experiences, and the consequences of use outside of the rave and gay circuit party settings remain limited. Several researchers have reported on negative experiences while using ecstasy (Baggot, 2002; Carlson et al., 2004; McElrath and McEvoy, 2002; Parrott et al., 2002). They portray users in terms of the number of pills taken in a designated amount of time, and associate amount of use with reported negative consequences, such as memory loss and depression. Carlson (2004) suggests that focusing on negative short- and long-term consequences could provide the basis for prevention programming with respect to a drug for which there are relatively few immediately observable unpleasant side effects. Baggot (2002) argues for a prevention strategy concentrating on some of the commonly reported adverse experiences, for example, those associated with binge use. Other researchers have reported on the misinformation that users receive and share with others, which may or may not lead to experimentation and use (McElrath and McEvoy, 2001). Only a handful of researchers have mentioned any association between ecstasy and sexuality (Zemishlany, Aizenberg, and Weizman, 2001). Several researchers have argued that there is no direct connection between ecstasy and sexual risk-taking (Beck and Rosenbaum, 1994). Others suggest that simultaneous use of ecstasy and alcohol has a greater effect on sexual behavior than ecstasy alone (Carlson, Falck, McCaughan, and Siegal, 2004; Sterk, Elifson, Theall, Greene, and Boeri, 2001). Additionally, the opportunities or pressures inherent in particular settings can significantly affect whether, under the influence of ecstasy, sexual risk-taking occurs or does not. On the other hand, there is substantial literature highlighting the association of ecstasy and risky sex among gay and bisexual men, especially club and circuit party attendees, mainly with respect to unprotected anal sex. For this group, ecstasy, as well as methamphetamine, are clearly disinhibitors, working in a variety of ways to increase sexual risk, especially among younger men and those who have recently "come out" (Klitzman, Greenberg, Pollack, and Dolezal, 2002; Mattison, Ross, Wolfson, and Franklin, 2001).

If there is little written about the social context and social use of ecstasy in general, there is even less information available about ecstasy use among inner city adolescents and young adults. For many of these youths, the rave or electronic dance environments are not typical. Though the use of the Internet is popular among inner city youth for playing games, our research has found that it is not widely used by this population as a source of drug information. Thus, knowledge of ecstasy use, adulterants, and protection against consequences are mainly obtained through personal networks, and in order to learn about inner city adolescents' and young adults' understanding of these topics and experiences with ecstasy, one must talk directly with them.

In 1999, in the context of another study on poly-drug use among inner city young adults, our research team identified ecstasy as a new drug in the Hartford club environment. Of the 401 individuals who completed our baseline survey between 1999 and 2001, 39% reported that they had ever used ecstasy, and 28% reported that they had used ecstasy in last 30 days. Ecstasy was diffused through inner city, primarily Puerto Rican, club attendees into inner city networks of users and eventually into existing street distribution systems (Schensul, 2001; Schensul et al., in this publication). Between 2000 and 2001, we were able to interview a number of ecstasy-using young adults about their use. This paper examines their encounters with ecstasy and their perceptions of the drug. More specifically, we will discuss initiation and setting; experiences on ecstasy; patterns of use; heavy users; pill ingredients; drug-mixing behaviors and attitudes; and perceptions of risks.

METHODS

This study was conducted as a supplement to a larger study of poly-drug use among inner city African-American and Puerto Rican adolescents and young adults between the ages of 16 and 24 (*Pathways to High Risk Drug Use Among Urban Youth*, NIDA Grant #R01-DA-11421, PI, J. Schensul; OAR supplement #DA-11421-02S1). It was conducted during the period 1999-2002 in low-income neighborhoods of Hartford, a poor mid-sized city of approximately 130,000 in the northeastern United States. The project was carried out through a partnership between the Institute for Community Research and the Hispanic Health Council. The purpose of the study was to identify multiple drug use trajectories, and to test the relative importance of vulnerability and social networks to contributing to differential drug use and pathways to hard drug use (Schensul and Burkholder, in press). The supplement's objectives were to explore the introduction of designer/club drugs into this inner city environment, document the meanings and use of club drugs, especially ecstasy, and describe the behaviors, consequences, and possible HIV risks associated with the use of these drugs. The interview data reported on here were obtained through the implementation of this supplement.

To explore the use of ecstasy in our inner city study population, we recruited 23 individuals for in-depth interviews. To obtain a sufficient number of in-depth interviews with key informants, we sought participants from the parent study who reported having used ecstasy and conducted additional recruitment through interviewees' peer groups and in local dance clubs and after-hours clubs. Accordingly, 18 of the participants were participants in the parent study, and five were not. Thirteen of the participants were male and 10 were female. The average age of the participants was 21-years-old, with a range from 17-24 years. Most of the participants were Puerto Rican, largely because at the time of the study, Puerto Ricans were much more likely to use ecstasy than other ethnic minority groups in Hartford. Five of the women identified themselves as bisexual or lesbian or discussed sex with other women, while none of the men identified themselves as anything other than heterosexual or discussed sex with other men. The participants had diverse social identities, which included raver, hip hop rapper, mother, honor roll student, party promoter, dancer, drug dealer, among others. The research team used four semi-structured interview guides which focused on club drug use, especially ecstasy and sexual behavior while using drugs; sexual history; knowledge about drug use and selling in local dance clubs, after-hour clubs, and raves; and STDs. All of the interviewees were asked questions from the guide about club drug use, and one of the three other guides, depending on their knowledge base and experience. Most interviews lasted close to two hours. Four of the participants were interviewed a second time. The participants were compensated $20 for each interview session.

INITIATION AND SETTING

The majority of the participants reported hearing about ecstasy from their friends. Many said that they had heard so many good things about it, that they wanted to try it. For example, Joseph, a 24-year-old African-American male, explained his first use by saying: "I just got curious about it. And then one day I went there (to an underground rave), [and] this dude was asking me if I knew anybody that wanted some ecstasy. I was [said], 'Yeah me!,' and I bought some, . . . and I tried it." Orlando, a 17-year-old African-American male, reported:

. . . What was it that really made me [try ecstasy]? Oh, it was . . . [hearing], "If you take a pill, and . . . you get a massage, you feel it throughout your whole body! It's . . . a real central feeling!" So I was like, "Word! I'm gonna try it! I'm gonna try it!"

He and his best friend now refer to it as "the Happy Pill." Other participants said that they had heard it was good for sex and would make them feel sexually aroused. For example, Alejandro, a 21-year-old Puerto Rican male, reported:

This girl [who was using ecstasy, that] I knew, came up to me [in the after-hours club]. . . . And she was like, . . . "You don't know about the 'E' thing?" I said, "Gets you mad horny!" I liked the girl. And then she gave me a half a pill . . . and then she was touching me.

Many of the participants said that initially they had received it for free from a friend. In some cases, the friend actually sold ecstasy; in other cases, a friend simply had bought multiple pills and felt like sharing them. Oleos, a 22-year-old Puerto Rican male, described "sharing ecstasy" in this way:

. . . I was not selling, but I was selling. . . . I used to be the one that used to [say], "Don't worry. I got you." I used to go to the . . . [the seller], bring them the money . . . I felt so good off this pill that I wanted everybody just to do it. If I had enough money to [pay for it for them], I would [pay for it] . . . 'cause I felt like this is the best thing that ever happened to me.

Only a few mentioned being introduced to ecstasy by dealers or users whom they did not know, and in these cases the participants were in a club at the time.

Participants' initial experience with ecstasy occurred in a range of locations, including regular-hour clubs, including hip hop, Latin, or techno, or after-hour clubs; raves; motels (a social venue for many of the participants in our larger Pathways sample); their own home or a friend's home; and even a psychiatric hospital. Salvador, a 24-year-old, Puerto Rican male, who was introduced to ecstasy in a regular-hours club, explained:

> The first time I tried ecstasy, two girls introduced it to me, and they were at it already, by the look on their face. And I was like, "Hey! How are ya feeling?" And they told me . . . they felt as if they were on a roller coaster with a bunch of butterflies in their stomach, and they asked me if I wanted to try it.

Although ecstasy use is common within the rave scene, only a small number of the participants said that they frequently go to raves; many more said that they frequently go to regular-hour dance clubs or after-hours clubs. The raves are special events with all-night music and dancing (Eiserman, Singer, Schensul, and Broomhall, 2003). They ban alcohol and allow access to minors. The after-hours are dance clubs that are usually open from about midnight into the early morning hours, do not serve alcohol, and may allow access to minors (Huebner, Singer, Schensul, Eiserman, and Burkholder, 2001). Attendees at both of these types of locations are mainly under 30 years of age and often substitute drug use for alcohol use. The lack of popularity of the raves among our participants is probably due in part to the high cost of entrance fees for raves as compared to the entrance fees associated with the regular clubs or after-hours clubs.

As is common with ecstasy use among other groups, the participants in our sample reported that most ecstasy use occurred at night and especially on the weekend nights while partying. After initial exposure, regular-hour and after-hours clubs, which all include dance music, seemed to be especially common sites for ecstasy use. The popularity of the after-hours clubs among our participants seems to be associated with the following factors: users tended to take the drug at night; the high they experienced reportedly lasted as long as six-to-eight hours, and users needed a place to go while they were still high and very much awake. The after-hours clubs also provided ready access to ecstasy pills, through individual dealers or through dealers who were affiliated with the clubs. The more often the participant reported having used ecstasy in her or his life, the more varied and plentiful was the list of reported venues and times at which s(he) reported having used it. In addition, participants, who used it most heavily, seemed to incorporate it into everyday activities over time, as opposed to infrequent or occasional users who used it mostly within the club setting. For example, Madalin, a 22-year-old Puerto Rican, who reportedly had used ecstasy around 200 times, described the sites in which she used the drug in this way:

I started doing it in the street every day. . . . Wherever I was. . . . Behind [the park] there's a big old parking lot. . . .You can hear the music from the club. . . . We used to just stand out there [while we were on ecstasy], put the car music on, and have fun.

Participants consistently described ecstasy as a "social" drug. For example, Nia, a 21-year-old Puerto Rican female, said, ". . . You don't wanna be alone when you're on ecstasy. You wanna be around people." Madalin explained:

. . . If you do it by yourself . . . Well, I tried it one time by myself in my house, and it was like the worst. Because you're in the house, and you just want to be outside around people and loud music. . . . You go crazy. You start hearing things. . . . I had to leave. I went outside, and I found my friends, and I was like, "I don't like being in the house." When I'm high [on E], I can't be in the house.

Ecstasy use, after initiation, was often a planned decision between two or more friends or significant others, and almost always included some type of social activity, e.g., going to a club, house party or motel, or having a one-on-one experience. Ecstasy usually triggers a desire within users, which can only be satisfied by other people, the desire to share and be emotionally and physically intimate, though not necessarily sexual. Participants also emphasized the urge to take it around boyfriends or girlfriends, or people who they were attracted to. Ideally, a person will experience an ecstasy high with other people who also are using the drug, and who can understand how s(he) is feeling and share the intense "ecstasy high" with her or him. Roberto, a 19-year-old Puerto Rican male, said, "You wanna be in an environment where there are people . . . that are in your same vibe, or . . . you wanna just be alone with your girl!" Finally, despite the feelings of openness and friendliness generated by ecstasy, participants preferred using the drug with people who they knew and trusted, rather than strangers. Salvador stated:

You really got to use it with people you trust. . . . You can't just do [it] with somebody you just met. Who knows [how] they can take advantage of you? They can say they popped it [the pill, and] they don't pop it. . . . They could just rob you. . . . They [could] dig in your pockets, knock you out, [and] you [couldn't] do nothing. . . .

EXPERIENCES ON ECSTASY

Most of the participants reported having multiple positive experiences with ecstasy. Many participants described feelings of happiness. Antonio, a 19-year-old Puerto Rican male, shared, "[On ecstasy,] I was feeling high, happy, rejoiceful . . . You feel good about yourself. It's a feeling that you never had before!" Alejandro said, "With the 'E' pill, you . . . get like, wow, loose and stuff . . . ! You're really happy, and then you want to be with a girl!" Roberto said that he used ecstasy to change his emotional state when he was feeling bad. Talking about one of the times he had used ecstasy, Roberto stated, ". . . I was upset and everything, and I just wanted to chill, . . . so I just did [ecstasy with my girlfriend]. I took it, like just to be happy for the first time in weeks. . . ."

Many participants also said that ecstasy gave them energy and made them feel like moving; consequently, they often liked to dance while using ecstasy. In this regard, Nia explained how one is able to tell who is using ecstasy in a club:

> . . . Let's say you get to the club at ten o'clock, nine o'clock, right? And you see the same person on the dance floor 'til fuckin' four, five o'clock in the morning. Then they gotta be on something! And they're all energetic and jumping around all night 'cause that's what ecstasy does. It hypes you up! It gives you energy! You be up all night!

Participants consistently reported enjoying the sensation-enhancing aspects of the drug. They mentioned that ecstasy positively affected sight, hearing, touch, and smell. Carlos, a 24-year-old Puerto Rican male, said, "All my senses were enhanced. You know, everything smelled good . . . . Everything felt different. It felt better." Only one person mentioned that ecstasy had a positive effect on taste. Roberto said that he liked to drink orange juice when he was high on ecstasy because "it tastes really good." Participants often recounted experiencing lights, music, and physical touch with another person in a different and much more powerful way when on the drug. Marco, a 17-year-old Puerto Rican male, explained:

> . . . It heightens your senses, heightens your touch, everything, you seem to see things, like colors, brighter. . . . But the feeling . . . to me, most of the high is just feeling . . . like when you get touched . . . !

Maritza, a 19-year-old, who self-identified as Cuban and Spanish, described ecstasy in this way:

> It was just incredible.... It was a beautiful high.... We were ... just getting ready to go to the club. The pill is kicking in, and I have one of my boys massaging my temples, I have another one massaging my hands, and another one massaging my feet, ... and it's just hitting me full force!

Joseph stated that, while under the influence of ecstasy, even the vibrations from the speakers in the club had an effect on him and enhanced his physical experience.

The participants also discussed objects or products that they used to enhance their sensory experience while on ecstasy. These items appear to be most commonly used in the dance club setting. Glow sticks are used as a form of entertainment and play for ecstasy users. Participants also talked about sniffing or inhaling Vicks VapoRub® nasal sticks, including individuals holding the substance near a user's face and blowing it towards them. Users reported that the vapors from this medicine increased their high on the drug. The menthol in the medication stimulates dilated bronchi, thereby enhancing the effect of the ecstasy (http://www.dea.gov/pubs/intel/01008). Some users even used surgical masks or gas masks lined with the substance to increase their high. A few participants also referred to drinking orange juice to enhance their high. Users also explained that when they are high on ecstasy, they feel the need to grind (bruxism, in medical terminology) or clench their teeth. Participants talked about sucking on lollipops or pacifiers, chewing gum and smoking cigarettes, while using ecstasy, to help alleviate these unpleasant (albeit tolerated) side effects (Arrue, Gomez, and Giralt, 2004).

The most sought after sensation-enhancing effect was touch. Exchange of massages and other types of touching were commonly described, even among strangers. For example, Nia said that she can tell when people, "especially girls," are on ecstasy because "they get real touchy-feely, and wanna be touched, like, 'Oh, hook me up with a massage!'" Accordingly, Barbara, a 22-year-old White female, talked about group massages in raves, referring to them as "E Trains": ". . . Everyone's on E, and they all sit in front of each other [giving the person in front of them a massage], like a massage train. . . ." For some, the combined experience of feeling the beat of the music and physical touch while rolling was highly erotic. Joseph, for example, described his experience with ecstasy in this way:

> . . . Things that in no way [you] would receive as sexual, when you're sober, when you do "E," you feel it sexually, even the pump of the music, the music touching your body, the people touching you. . . . Everything that . . . different people experience within themselves just turns sexual.

The majority of the participants discussed physically affectionate exchanges between friends, lovers, or new acquaintances, while on ecstasy, which may or may not have led to sex. Damaris, a 22-year-old Puerto Rican female, explained her experience this way:

> . . . You do so many things that you wouldn't do, when you're not on it. You . . . flirt with people that you're with, and you won't even recognize that's what you are doing. . . . People [have] come up to us and start[ed] doing stuff that you would never think that they would do, . . . and you . . . respond back to them. Like, they . . . come up to you and kiss you without even knowing you, or start touching you. But you['re] so high, that you go with the flow. . . .

Many participants also described ecstasy as a sexual enhancer, since it both increased sexual desire and magnified the positive experience of touch. For example, Madalin said, "Ecstasy . . . will make me feel horny, like they touch me, and it feels so good. . . . You want to have sex when you're on ecstasy . . ." Consequently, of the 23 interviewees, 17 reported having had sexual intercourse on ecstasy. Of the remaining six, one was a virgin, but reported that she had numerous non-penetrative sexual experiences on ecstasy. Some participants described using ecstasy specifically to loosen their inhibitions and to facilitate sexual experimentation. For example, Olga, an 18-year-old Puerto Rican female, told the following story:

> The first time I did it . . . it was with my boyfriend and my [female] friend, and I was having a threesome. So we were like, "Let's see if the E will really get us there," 'cause I really don't like girls. . . . We bought E. . . . We popped them. After like 15 minutes, I was like, "Hi." My best friend was touching my back. . . . And one thing led to another. Then we was all three of us having sex. . . .

Many participants reported that their sexual experiences lasted longer on ecstasy and that, because of this, sex was improved by ecstasy use. The length of sexual interludes seemed to be related to difficulties obtaining erections and experiencing orgasms. Both male and female participants reported that, while using ecstasy, males at times took longer to get an erection, and regularly took longer to ejaculate. Females did not report any problems with arousal or orgasm. A few of the women mentioned that using ecstasy with a male lover can be a challenge because both partners usually do not peak on the drug or become aroused at the same time.

Most negative experiences during ecstasy use seemed to be associated with using too many pills at once, getting a "bad" pill (one which had effects that they did not enjoy), or using "E" simultaneously with certain other drugs. Accordingly, given that participants so regularly used ecstasy with other drugs, it was often difficult to determine which drug, if any, was more responsible for the bad experience. For example, Damaris shared a story about an unsettling situation that occurred after she had mixed ecstasy with other drugs:

> ... We was all drinking, and most of 'em were on the "E" pill, and most of 'em were just getting high off weed, and whatever else. . . . The next day I woke up with such a headache, and I couldn't remember parts of the party. . . . And they come and tell me, "You know, you ended up, you and [your] mother-in-law was like taking your clothes off . . . and they had to stop y'all." And I'm like, "No. I'm not that kind of person. . . ." And I couldn't remember. . . .

In terms of side effects, nausea and throwing up were the most commonly reported. While only a few of the participants actually reported having thrown up themselves, a number of them mentioned knowing someone else who regularly threw up after taking it. Interestingly, they reported that they and their friends continued to use ecstasy, even though it had this effect on them. For example, Antonio said that he sometimes throws up after first ingesting the pill, but that he still uses it because he enjoys the high so much.

The degree of negativity associated with the aftereffects of ecstasy use varies from person to person. Many users reported feeling very tired after coming down from an ecstasy high. Of course, this was usually after they had stayed up all night, using ecstasy and partying. While some users reported also feeling uncomfortable or irritable, having a lack of appetite, feeling down, or craving more ecstasy, others did not mention these types of negative aftereffects. As one might expect, the heaviest ecstasy users were most apt to emphasize these effects in their interviews. For example, Julia, a 24-year-old Puerto Rican female, said, ". . . I noticed that I didn't like the morning after. . . . [I felt] shitty. I was dehydrated. I just wanted to sleep all day. . . . I just couldn't eat anything . . . for . . . the whole next day. . . ." Still, it seems that these effects were not unpleasant enough to cause participants to change their use patterns, until after many episodes of use.

Only two of the 23 participants, Enrique, a 17-year-old Puerto Rican male, and Ellie, a 24-year-old Puerto Rican female, reported not liking ecstasy. They both said that they never wanted to do it again. Enrique reported that he had only used it once and had felt like he was "flipping out." Ellie explained her experiences with ecstasy in this way:

> . . . It was real funny. My whole body was numb. I felt like I wanted to run, fly, scream, have sex, do everything. Then I felt sleepy, but I couldn't sleep. . . . It stayed in my body for two days. I couldn't eat. I couldn't sleep. I couldn't do nothing, just stay stuck like a fiend the next day. . . . I did it twice, and then the next month, I did it two more times. And then I said, 'This shit ain't for me. . . .' It's the feeling the next day . . . . You don't want to get up from the bed. Once you close your eyes, you won't get up for like 10 hours, and you feel like shit. . . !

Ellie went on to say that the last time that she used ecstasy, she also used cocaine and got into a knife fight with another girl. It seemed that this event may have contributed to her disinterest in using ecstasy again. Only one other participant, Olga, mentioned engaging in violence while under the influence of ecstasy. Olga said that prior to the second time that she used ecstasy, she had been angry with her boyfriend. After they took the pill, they had gotten in a fight, in which she broke his car window and ended up in jail. Despite this, as soon as she was released from jail, she and her boyfriend started drinking and using ecstasy again. Based on our findings, few participants had negative experiences while using ecstasy, other than an isolated incident or two, but a number of them, mostly all heavier users, discussed negative aftereffects associated with prolonged use.

PATTERNS OF USE

Reported occasions of use among the participants varied from one time to over 200 times. There were three main use patterns among participants: infrequent user (experimenters who had used ecstasy no more than 4-6 times during their lifetime); occasional user (about 10 to 20 times during their lifetime); and heavy user (40 times or more; multiple times every week or weekend for a period of time). Participants reported using anywhere between a half of a pill and four pills at a time. Some mentioned using only a half a pill the first time, in order to test out how sensitive they were to the drug. This was a technique utilized after the first time as well, when the user had determined s(he) was sensitive to ecstasy or when s(he) thought that s(he) had received a very strong pill. Participants reported that sometimes they ingested multiple pills during a night, in order to maintain their high over many hours.

Users who discussed why they did not use ecstasy more regularly, usually pointed to cost or access as the reason. At the time of the study (2000-2001), the pill could generally be obtained on an individual basis in Hartford for about $20 dollars on the street or in clubs. This price was considered exorbitant to many members of the sample, who were of lower economic status. Carla, a 22-year-old female, who identified as Indian, Latina and African-American, said, ". . . It made me feel nice, but that's not something I would want to do again. Maybe it's because it costs $20, and I will not spend $20 for a pill." Some users talked about their future use of ecstasy, as being wholly dependent on when they could obtain the drug for free from a friend who was more economically stable or who was a drug seller. Based on the reports of the participants, the desire to use ecstasy with others, as opposed to using it alone, was so great that it was not uncommon for a friend to pay for multiple pills themselves to share with other friends. One participant, Carlos, explained that he was living on the street and sniffing heroin every day, so he was only able to use ecstasy when his friend bought it for him. A few of the users reported cutting way back or even stopping their use of ecstasy once the drug was no longer easily accessible to them. Sonia, a 21-year-old Puerto Rican female, had been a regular user for a number of months, but within the six months prior to the interview, had used it only once. She explained:

> . . . I used to do it a lot in the summer. I used to [do] it like every weekend. And then I stopped talking to that guy [that I was dating who gave it to me], so I don't really do it. . . . I've been wanting to do it. . . . It's just kind of hard to find. It's not like you could walk up to somebody in the streets, "Hey, you got [E]?. . . ." The thing about it is, I never paid for it. . . . It's twenty dollars, twenty-five dollars. I don't want it that badly. . . . If I want to go to the club, and

I want to do it, then I'll pay for it. But I never pay for it, so [I] be like, "Damn, twenty dollars for one pill is kind of a lot!"

A number of the participants were currently or had been drug dealers in the past, which explained how they could afford to pay for it and share it with others. Gio, an 18-year-old Puerto Rican male; Oleos; Barbara; and Salvador reported that they had been ecstasy dealers, or were currently ecstasy dealers. Madalin said that she was able to afford ecstasy because she was a heroin dealer, which was fairly lucrative.

HEAVY USERS

There were six individuals, one male and five females, who could clearly be designated as having been heavy users at one point or another. In the case of the heavy users, once they tried it, they began using it heavily (at least every week) fairly quickly, within a few weeks or months. Olga, for example, reported that she had used ecstasy about 90 times during the month of October 1999, "three pills every day." Olga said that she and a female lover would always do it together. When her boyfriend found out about the affair and the ecstasy use, he broke up with her. She stopped using ecstasy regularly at that point; she had used ecstasy only twice in the nine months prior to the interview. Omar, a 21-year-old Puerto Rican male, reported having used it about 75 times over five months, "only on weekends" at first, and then "every other day and the whole weekend." He said that he had slowed down his use recently because he "took three pills [at the same time] and [his] high didn't . . . go away for two days, and [he] got scared."

Notably, periods of particularly heavy use led to efforts to stop using ecstasy or at least cut down on use, as the negative effects began to intensify. Many heavy users stopped using regularly because they no longer felt as good on the drug as when they initially had started. For example, Maritza said that she started using ecstasy in March of 2000 and then used it about 90 times over the following seven months; initially every three weeks, and then "every day." She explained:

. . . I would pop a pill [at] . . . one o'clock in the morning, two o'clock in the morning. . . . I would be in the club until five [o'clock] the next morning. . . . So the [next] night, I [would] be just coming down [from "E" at] like around ten-thirty, eleven o'clock, and I [would] pop another pill. . . . It was a constant high for me. . . .

Maritza said that over time, her ecstasy use "was slowly but surely just fading." She described the experience as the following:

> . . . It wasn't even attractive to me any more. . . . I started feeling disgusted about it. It was just the way it made me feel. The way my jaw would lock, . . . so I couldn't even talk. And just the way, being in the clubs, and the lights, and the way your head feels. . . . At the very beginning, it was like, "Woo hoo! Let's do some more." But after a while, . . . I started not liking it anymore. It was just like the worst time in my life . . . the worst high. It was just like, "Why am I doing it?" because it wasn't a happy high. . . . I would just sit there and be a grump.

Other heavy users also talked about this feeling of "burn out," which set in after one too many intense experiences on ecstasy, one too many late nights, and one too many days spent feeling tired, irritable, and/or depressed after a night or weekend of use.

In August of 2000, Maritza was involved in a serious car accident, in which she was thrown from the car and broke three ribs and received 10 staples in her head. After that incident, she stopped using all drugs, including ecstasy. At the time of the interview, Maritza had not used ecstasy at all for six months. She said that it "was just basically a test for myself, and I proved myself right that I can stop when I want to stop, and a lot of people didn't think I was able to do that."

Julia, one of Maritza's best friends, said that she had used ecstasy about 40 times over 10 months; it was a "Thursday through Sunday thing, sometimes on a Monday, Tuesday, or Wednesday." Julia said that she continued to use ecstasy regularly for about three months after the time that Maritza stopped. She said that in the last three months prior to the interview, she had been using ecstasy "once in a blue moon, on the weekends." She explained that she had not liked the aftereffects of ecstasy, was concerned about addiction, and decided to stop using as part of a pact with Maritza: " 'Cause me and my friend, we kinda made a promise that we weren't gonna to do it so heavily. . . ." Another participant, Madalin, said that she used ecstasy about 200 times over seven months, "every day." She said that she decided to quit using ecstasy a month before the interview out of a concern about loss of weight, insomnia, and a fear of addiction.

Heavy users found that over time they had to increase the number of pills that they took simultaneously or take more over a number of hours to get the same effect. Barbara, a 22-year-old White female, who reported having used ecstasy more than 200 times over four years, said she had decided to stop using ecstasy two months before the interview, and that one of the reasons for this was because she was not experiencing the same effect from the drug that she had before. It appears that, as with known addictive drugs, like heroin, tolerance of ecstasy appears to develop after repeated use, leading to increases in frequency of use. However, only a small number of users in our sample followed this pattern. It may be that the cost of ecstasy reduces the likelihood that most users of lower economic status are able to use ecstasy enough to develop a tolerance.

Heavy users who had used ecstasy compulsively for some period of time, were the only interviewees, besides the two participants who had tried ecstasy and quickly decided that they did not like it, who mentioned having voluntarily stopped or changed the frequency of their ecstasy use. However, given that only a short period of time had passed since their last period of regular use, it was unclear at the time of the interviews whether these users would in fact be able to maintain a more infrequent use pattern.

PILL INGREDIENTS

More experienced (occasional and heavy) ecstasy users were aware that MDMA is usually combined with other illicit drugs or fillers to make ecstasy pills, in order to increase manufacturers' and dealers' profit margin. Ecstasy, unlike many other pills, comes in various widths and lengths, and colors. The pills usually have symbols on them, and are named according to these symbols. Accordingly, ecstasy pills can vary greatly in purity, as well as in the other ingredients, including other psychoactive drugs or even noxious substances (Singer, in press). Barbara explained: ". . . The pills just weren't as good as they used to be. . . . I think they were just bad pills. There was just too much filler, not enough ecstasy, not enough MDMA. . . ." Users over time will come to know that certain pills are stronger or yield a better high and will seek out the dealer who they know has access to those pills. For example, Julia explained:

> I got one that I didn't like, and that to me, is considered a bad high.
> I don't remember what it was called, but it was the shape of a heart
> and a pink color. . . . It was just more of a dopey feeling. You know
> how dope (heroin) makes you kinda . . . in la-la land. . . . It wasn't
> more of that upbeat type of high that you usually get.

Sonia said that her only bad experience on ecstasy had been one time when she had taken a pill, called "X Files," which she had heard was a particularly strong kind of ecstasy. She said that after she took the pill, she had hallucinated, had problems seeing, and felt that her mouth was numb and that she could not move it.

Some participants variously categorized ecstasy pills as being stimulants, depressants, or hallucinogens depending on their effects. This division seems to coincide with street mythology that many ecstasy pills also have heroin, cocaine, or LSD in them. When asked if she knew what ecstasy was cut with, Olga said, "They told me dope (heroin), cocaine, and baking soda." Barbara added:

> If you look at the pill, and it has a lot of brown dots on it, that's heroin, or if you have a pill that's colored, a lot of times that has heroin in it too. They just dye it so that you can't really tell as much. You definitely know if you take it. If it's speedy, you're just going to be up and wired. If it's got a lot of heroin in it, you're going to be a little more relaxed. . . .

A few participants reported that pills with heroin in it will make the user throw up. In fact, the organization, EcstasyData.org directs a laboratory testing program of "ecstasy" pills obtained from users from across the United States. In collaboration with DanceSafe, MAPS (The Multidisciplinary Association for Psychedelic Studies), Erowid, and the Promind Foundation, they have been doing lab testing of ecstasy pills since 1996 (http://www.ecstasydata.org/about.php). EctasyData. org has not found heroin or LSD in any of the 807 "ecstasy" samples that have been sent to them (http://www.ecstasydata.org/datastats.php). Furthermore, they only have found cocaine in five pills. Two of these pills also contained MDMA.

Some of the more experienced ecstasy users did discuss the risk of getting bad pills, i.e., pills that are sold as ecstasy but are, actually, some other drug, combination of other drugs, or other substance(s) (and no MDMA). These users placed a high emphasis on knowing their sellers and, in turn, the quality product that s(he) was selling. The reason for this is that pure MDMA is an expensive chemical, and sellers will try to pass off other drugs which are cheaper, easier to manufacture, or more accessible than ecstasy, as ecstasy pills. Carla said that the second time that she used ecstasy:

It didn't really have an effect on me. . . . In fact, [I] came down really quick, before I even left the club. . . . Some people in the club were saying, "That's not the same 'X-Factor' that we had the last time in the club!," and that it was 'garbage.'

Unfortunately, some of these alternative pills have substances which are more dangerous to users than ecstasy itself, and the negative effects of the use of these drugs, including death, has at times contributed to the nationwide panic about ecstasy use (Singer, in press; Parrott, 2004).

DRUG MIXING BEHAVIORS AND ATTITUDES

Most participants reported that they used other drugs at the same time that they used ecstasy. The most commonly reported "other" drugs that were used simultaneously with ecstasy were marijuana and/or alcohol. In some cases, participants reported that the multi-drug use was simply a coincidence because they were introduced to ecstasy for the first time, after they had already ingested another drug. Some reported intentionally taking the drugs simultaneously because they liked the type of high that they experienced with the combination. Others reported taking marijuana after having taken an "E" pill hours earlier, in order to enhance the high that they were feeling, or get a "pick me up" when the effects of the drug had started to wane a bit. Others reported using other drugs as they were "coming down" off of "E," so that they felt better, i.e., did not experience the negative feelings sometimes associated with the period immediately following the ecstasy high. While combining ecstasy with other drugs would appear to be one of the biggest risks associated with ecstasy use, only a few participants expressed concern about drug interactions and overdoses, and most of these were after they had had a bad experience.

Many of the participants used marijuana on a daily basis and did not consider it to be a dangerous drug. As a result, their marijuana use seemed to be unrelated to their ecstasy use. Others talked about using ecstasy as way to feel a stronger high than what they experienced from marijuana use alone. Damaris explained that she never uses "E" alone. She said:

Well . . . when we do E is usually at night time, . . . [and] we been the whole day either smoking the weed already, since the morning time, and . . . maybe drinking. So . . . by the time we do the E pill, we so drunk and already high . . . from the weed, that the E pill is just a higher high for us. . . . 'Cause we smoke weed . . . every day, [and] . . . I been smoking weed for so long that . . . weed won't do anything for me. So maybe that's why we combine the weed and . . . the E pill . . .!

Marco said, "[When I use marijuana], it maintains the high. Sometimes when [I] start coming down from the high, sometimes I'll smoke a [marijuana] blunt, and it will bring it up a little bit."

Alcohol was used by participants mostly as a party drug, i.e., they would drink when they went to clubs or house parties. Alejandro explained that he always uses ecstasy and alcohol together. He stated:

. . . People always told me that it feels good with beer. It's something that you do. [People told me] to always do it with beer. And I don't know why.

While in the minority, a few participants mentioned reasons for not using ecstasy and alcohol simultaneously. Omar, a 21-year-old Puerto Rican male, said that while he uses marijuana with ecstasy, he does not use alcohol with it because "it takes your high away." Roberto said:

You can't drink on that [ecstasy]. . . . It messes up your whole groove. That's what I heard, so that's why I don't try it. . . . You know, your vibe, your groove, your mood. . . . The way you feel, it upsets your stomach. You just want to throw up. . . . I heard it brings you[r high] down too!

Ellie also said that she tried drinking alcohol with the pill and found "that you can't get drunk on ecstasy." Sonia said that she does not use any other drugs, especially alcohol, on "E" because "they say when you're on [it], that you shouldn't mix liquor . . . because you could die or you could have an overdose. You could have a bad trip. So I don't. . . ." Maritza said that "If you drink alcohol on it (E), it can be fatal." Salvador said, ". . . Some say it's not good, taking pills with alcohol, so you gotta watch that!" However, a few of the participants, who repeated these warnings, had used alcohol and ecstasy at the same time. Only one participant made the link between alcohol and dehydration. Madalin said that alcohol dehydrates you, so she "only drinks one or two beers when on ecstasy." It is unclear why there were so many contradictory perceptions about combining alcohol and ecstasy among our sample.

One possibility is that information which takes a clear stand on the level of risk associated with mixing alcohol and ecstasy may not be available, or at least not available to this population.

Participants also mentioned using "dust" (embalming fluid with additives) (Singer, Juvalis, and Weeks, 2000; Singer et al., in press; Singer et al., this publication), LSD, mushrooms, crack cocaine, regular cocaine, heroin methamphetamine, PCP, and over-the-counter stimulants, e.g., No Doz, while under the influence of ecstasy. Not surprisingly, when asked about bad experiences on ecstasy, participants most often mentioned experiences in which they had used three or more drugs. Julia talked about one occasion that she had used four pills, "dust," marijuana, and alcohol, and was outside in hot summer weather at a crowded parade in New York City. She said that she had felt wobbly, numb, and nauseous, and eventually passed out. Surprisingly, only Madalin expressed any concern about overdosing from using too many pills or mixing ecstasy with other drugs, like "dust." She said:

> I don't recommend people doing "E" and dust at the same time. . . . People die like that, you know, you get so high, you don't know what you're doing. You be fighting with people, and you don't even know why you fighting.

PERCEPTIONS OF RISKS

Despite all of the public health and media attention that has been focused on drug use, in general, participants did not seem overly concerned about the risks of ecstasy use. As we saw in the prior sections on pill ingredients and mixing, some were aware of the dangers, and attempted to reduce their risks. Some participants emphasized the need to drink water, suggesting that they were aware of the risk of dehydration. Roberto said, "[When you're on ecstasy,] you be drinking mad water. . . . You always thirsty, like you ran a mile!" Most users' perceptions about health risks seemed to come from their own personal experiences or from other users whom they knew. For example, Maritza experienced both weight loss and insomnia during the period that she frequently used ecstasy. Maritza explained:

> I lost weight. I wasn't eating right. I was very agitated. You couldn't tell me anything. I would rip your head off in a matter of 2.2 seconds. . . . Because with the ecstasy, you don't want to eat. . . . I

would be in the club until five [o'clock] the next morning. I would go home, catch maybe an hour sleep, [then] I would wake up. . . .

Madalin also said that she had lost too much weight while using ecstasy, and that when she was using ecstasy regularly, she was down to 100 lbs. and "really skinny." She said that when she was using as much as five pills a day, she would be high for two days straight "with no sleeping, no eating, just drinking water and orange juice." Julia explained: "I just didn't like what it would do to my body. . . ."

Madalin also expressed a concern about the possibility of addiction as follows: ". . . You get addicted to it. . . . I think it's the mind, but it's confusing because your body wants it. It is like you wanna feel like that . . . and you really have to get it!" Julia said that she had stopped using ecstasy heavily because ". . . I just didn't want to see myself getting hooked." Maritza, another former heavy user, mentioned knowing ecstasy users who had entered drug treatment in order to stop using. She said:

> The younger generation, like my age bracket, [up to age] 25, have tried ecstasy, and some have gotten to the point where they have needed rehab for it. And some have been able, like myself, to take it, when they want to, and stop when they want to. They just have that will power. Others haven't been able to. I have family members . . . [and] . . . a couple of friends that went to rehab for ecstasy.

Others described risks consequences having to do with the sexual effects of the drug. Nia said:

> . . . It can be dangerous and risky, if you're at a rave and you're a female, you're a young lady on ecstasy. Guys are going to try to take advantage of that . . . especially if they know you're on it because they think that you wanna have sex right away. So that's why you have to be careful, especially if you're hanging out with a guy.

A couple of participants specifically mentioned having received public health warnings about ecstasy from documentaries. Sonia described what she learned from watching a documentary on MTV:

> . . . There was this girl, and they did a cat scan on her head, and she had huge holes in her head. . . . Then they say, after a long time of

use, 'cause I guess it takes out a certain chemical from your brain that . . . alters your mood, like whether you're happy. . . . So . . . people need to get on medication because they don't have that chemical. . . . So they have to be put on anti-depressants because they become really depressed. But I don't do it like . . . that's people who did it hardcore, like every day. . . . I just don't do it like that. Certain stuff like that scares me, or like you hear someone dies in the club, and . . . they thought it was ecstasy pills, but it [was] something else, and the [person's] body burned out and [the person] died. . . . Like this thing in Florida . . . that you don't really touch people's ecstasy, and if [it] comes [in] certain colors, then it doesn't have [that drug] in it. [But] some people still take it. They're crazy . . . !

The drug that Sonia was referring to that was responsible for this and other similar deaths, is called "PMA," a drug which initially gives users a high reminiscent of ecstasy, but causes users' temperatures to raise to lethal levels (Singer, in press). Although Sonia did not stop using ecstasy after hearing this information, she said that not knowing what is in the pill has made her more selective about her sources for ecstasy. This, in turn, had contributed to a decrease in her use, because at the time of the interview she had not had much contact with her regular source, whom she trusted.

Barbara, a heavy poly-drug user, said that she was concerned about the effect of ecstasy, along with other drugs, on her memory. She explained: "I used to have a really good memory, and it's horrible now. That's one of the reasons why I stopped. . . ." One other participant mentioned concerns about ecstasy killing brain cells. Orlando said:

I know the dangers. . . . E kills brain cells. So, I'm thinking if it kills a certain amount of brain cells, and I've only done it two or three times, if I was to continue to do it, I wouldn't be left with too much.

He explained that he had learned this information from a card that he had received at a local rave from a girl who was under the influence of ecstasy at the time. When asked about how he thought this ironic situation had come about, he was unable to explain it. He simply said that some of the club goers were handing out fliers advertising other dance parties, and that the girl had probably felt like handing something out, and had found the cards somewhere and started giving them to people.

The general lack of public health information on ecstasy is best seen in the case of Reggie, a 19-year-old African-American male who, despite having had sex on ecstasy, expressed the following concern: ". . . It's [having sex while using E] probably not good for your body. If you're on drugs, it messes up your sperm cells. . . . [You] probably couldn't have no kid. But [I'm] just saying, I would do it. You understand? I would have sex with a girl, if I was on ecstasy, but I'd rather not." As these examples illustrate, however, concerns about potential long-term health risks did not stop these individuals from using ecstasy.

CONCLUSION

This study demonstrates that patterns of ecstasy use among inner city populations are shaped by the interaction of users with their social and cultural environment as well as the drug's availability and cost. For example, those users who were drug sellers or had close relationships with drug sellers seemed to have greater access to ecstasy as well as higher use patterns. In addition, the dance club, hip hop, Latin, or techno, and after-hour club settings seemed to be common environments for introduction to ecstasy and, especially, ecstasy use. Based on our research, it appears that the dance club and after-hours clubs represent the point of entry for ecstasy into the inner city: suburban, White adolescents and young adults who sold and/or used ecstasy came to Hartford clubs and mixed with inner city, mostly Latino and Black, adolescents and young adults. Still, many of the participants reported using ecstasy in other environments as well. The diversity of our study sample in terms of ethnicity, gender, social identity, and sexual orientation reflects the heterogeneous cultural environment of many mid- and large-sized cities in America. Although we did not recruit based on ethnicity, and there are fewer African-American residents than Latino residents in Hartford, the ethnic breakdown of our participants corresponds with national studies showing higher rates of ecstasy use among Latinos (particularly among Puerto Ricans) compared with African-Americans (Yacoubian, 2002).

Personal motivations for ecstasy use among our participants resemble those found in rave and other youth populations in America and elsewhere around the world. Ecstasy use is motivated by a desire to feel happy, to have increased energy, to facilitate social bonding and to enhance sensual pleasures of dancing, listening to music, touching and sex. However, virtually no mention is made of the "mind-opening" or spiritual awakening experiences common among ravers (Nencini, 2002; Reynolds, 1999). Ecstasy use within inner city settings appears to reflect values rooted in inner city party culture and street drug culture, as opposed to classic rave culture, which more closely resembled the psychedelic drug culture of the 1960s.

There was a general consensus among our participants that one should not use ecstasy when alone, since it is primarily a social drug. Ecstasy is mainly used in club and party settings or smaller social gatherings, where the desired social and sensual effects are enhanced. Cultural elements associated with raves, such as use of glow sticks and the giving of massages, have diffused into inner city nightclubs and after-hour settings, creating an environment which implicitly supports the use of ecstasy. Unlike the traditional raves, however, these environments have fewer protective mechanisms in place to prevent adverse outcomes. Most of the participants also seemed to have little information about ecstasy and other club drugs from publicly available sources, as compared to the few ravers in our sample, and ravers in general. Although bottled water is available, use of ecstasy with alcohol is common. Harm reduction organizations like DanceSafe, which provide free testing of ecstasy pills at raves, have little presence in these settings. In inner city club environments, ecstasy is commonly used to facilitate casual and anonymous sexual encounters, thus increasing the likelihood of engaging in sexual risk-taking behavior. Most ecstasy users in club and party environments are poly-drug users. In our sample, marijuana and alcohol are the most common drugs combined with ecstasy, followed by dust. This suggests that when certain types of drugs, e.g., club drugs, are introduced into inner city settings, they expand the drug repertoire and risks of drug mixing, rather than replacing commonly used drugs, as opposed to other drugs, e.g., crack cocaine, which became the drug of choice for certain individuals.

We observed a range of different frequencies of use, from infrequent to occasional to heavy. Equal numbers of our participants fell into each frequency of use category, i.e., about 7-8 people per category. The most frequent use took place on weekends, as this is the most popular time for clubbing and parties. The frequency of ecstasy use varied with the availability and cost of the drug. The more available and the lower the price of the drug, the more frequent the use and vice versa. Most users received ecstasy from friends, some of whom were dealers. It was not clear from our data where participants purchased the drug most often, but there was evidence of dealing occurring in and around clubs as well as in neighborhoods. Thus, relatively lower rates of ecstasy use within inner city populations compared with suburban populations may be due, in part, to lower access and higher cost of the drug relative to income bracket.

Most infrequent and occasional users reported fewer health risks and consequences from using the drug, compared with heavy users. Consistent with other research on MDMA, adverse events such as weight loss, depression, sleeplessness, hallucinations, vomiting and memory loss were reported. Additionally, there were several reports of participants feeling violent or angry, or lethargic (as a result of pills which had a "depressant" effect) while under the influence of the drug. Since most heavy ecstasy users were also poly-drug users, we cannot be sure that these adverse events are attributable to MDMA. While a number of experienced users suspected that their pills were adulterated, none of them actually reported having gotten their pills tested for MDMA; rather, they expected their "high" to vary depending upon the ingredients. Heavy use consistently led to "burn out," rather than long-term addiction. Heavy users reported that the effects of the high diminished after using it regularly, leading them eventually to stop taking the drug, particularly after experiencing an adverse event.

We did not find much evidence of permanent adverse effects from MDMA use among our participants. Consistent with other findings, ecstasy does not appear to be physically addictive. We have found evidence supporting the concept of "controlled drug use," since users tended to engage in distinct behaviors to manage (mostly enhance) the effects of the high and protect themselves from some adverse risks. More significantly, they appeared to be able to stop or reduce use at will. The greatest risk appears to stem from poly-drug use. Low levels of condom use generally, coupled with higher levels of sexual experimentation while using ecstasy, increase the risks of contracting STDs, including HIV.

These findings point to the need for more in-depth research on MDMA use within inner city settings, with a particular focus on ethnic and cultural context, self-controlled drug use, poly-drug mixing and sex risk behaviors. Further research is needed on how cultural norms and values within different inner city populations may influence different expectancies, attitudes, and use patterns of ecstasy. The concept of controlled drug use seems especially relevant to understanding patterns of ecstasy use, since it does not appear to be highly physically addictive, and the experience of detrimental aftereffects seems to surpass the feelings of psychological dependency over time. Since the risks of experiencing adverse events and consequences from ecstasy seem to increase with both quantity and frequency of use, researchers would benefit from greater consistency across clinical and non-clinical studies in defining these different levels. More research is also needed on the effects and consequences of combining MDMA with other drugs, especially marijuana and alcohol. Finally, the evidence of high levels of sexual experimentation, multiple-sex partners, and low levels of condom use in this population calls for further research on the relationship between ecstasy use and sex risk.

REFERENCES

Agar, M., and Reisinger, H. S. (2004). Ecstasy: Commodity or disease? *Journal of Psychoactive Drugs* 36 (2): 253-264.

Arria, A. M., Yacoubian, G. S., Jr., Fost, E., and Wish, E. D. (2002). The pediatric forum: Ecstasy use among club rave attendees. *Archives of Pediatrics and Adolescent Medicine* 156 (3): 295-296.

Arrue, A., Gomez, F. M., and Giralt, M. T. (2004). Effects of 3,4-methylenedioxymethamphetamine ('ecstasy') on the jaw-opening reflex and on the alpha(2)- adrenoceptors which regulate this reflex in the anesthetized rat. *European Journal of Oral Sciences* 112 (2): 127-133.

Baggot, M. J. (2002). Preventing problems in ecstasy users: Reduce use to reduce harm. *Journal of Psychoactive Drugs* 34 (2): 145-162.

Beck, J., and Rosenbaum, M. (1994). *Pursuit of ecstasy: The MDMA experience.* Albany: State University of New York Press.

Brewer, N. T. (2003). The relation of internet searching to club drug knowledge and attitudes. *Psychology and Health* 18: 387-401.

Carlson, R. G., Falck, R. S., McCaughan, J. A., and Siegal, H. A. (2004). MDMA/ecstasy use among young people in Ohio: Perceived risk and barriers to intervention. *Journal of Psychoactive Drugs* 36 (2): 181-189.

Carlson, R. G., McCaughan, J. A., Falck, R. S., Wang, J., Siegal, H. A., and Daniulaityte, R. (2004). Perceived adverse consequences associated with MDMA/Ecstasy use among young polydrug users in Ohio: Implications for intervention. *International Journal of Drug Policy* 15 (4): 265-274.

Diamond, S., Bermudez, R., and Schensul, J. (under review). What's the rap about ecstasy: Popular music lyrics and drug trends among American youth. *Journal of Adolescent Research.*

Eiserman, J. M., Singer, M., Schensul, J. J., and Broomhall, L. (2003). Methodological challenges in club drug research. *Practicing Anthropology* 25 (3): 19-22.

Falck, R. S., Carlson, R. G., Wang, J. C., and Siegal, H. A. (2004). Sources of information about MDMA (3, 4-methylenedioxymethamphetamine): Perceived accuracy, importance, and implications for prevention among young adult users. *Drug and Alcohol Dependence* 74 (1): 45-54.

Gross, S. R., Barrett, S. P., Shestowsky, J. S., and Pihl, R. O. (2002). Ecstasy and drug consumption patterns: A Canadian rave population study. *Canadian Journal of Psychiatry–Revue Canadienne de Psychiatrie* 47 (6): 546-551.

Haddad, P. M., Strickland, P., Anderson, I., Deakin, J. F., and Dursun, S. M. (2002). Effects of MDMA (ecstasy) use and abstention on serotonin neurons. *Lancet* 359 (9317): 1616-1618.

Hinchliff, S. (2001). The meaning of ecstasy use and clubbing to women in the late 1990's. *International Journal of Drug Policy* 12 (5-6): 455-468.

Hitzler, R. (2002). Pill kick: The pursuit of "ecstasy" at techno-events. *Journal of Drug Issues* 32 (2): 459-466.

Huebner, C., Singer, M., Schensul, J. J., Eiserman, J., and Burkholder, G. (2001). *Urban youth, 'club drugs,' and party culture.* Merida, Yucatan Mexico: The Society for Applied Anthropology Annual Meeting, March 28-31, Session F-75.

Johnston, L. D., O'Malley, P. M., and Bachman, J. G. (2003). Monitoring the future national results on adolescent drug use. Overview of key findings, 2002. In *NIH Publication No. 03-5374.* Bethesda: National Institute on Drug Abuse.

Klitzman, R. L., Greenberg, J. D., Pollack, L. M., and Dolezal, C. (2002). MDMA ('ecstasy') use, and its association with high risk behaviors, mental health, and other factors among gay/bisexual men in New York City. *Drug and Alcohol Dependence* 66 (2): 115-125.

Klitzman, R. L., Pope, H. G., Jr., and Hudson, J. I. (2000). MDMA ("Ecstasy") abuse and high-risk sexual behaviors among 169 gay and bisexual men. *American Journal of Psychiatry* 157 (7): 1162-1164.

Lee, S. J., Galanter, M., Dermatis, H., and McDowell, D. (2003). Circuit parties and patterns of drug use in a subset of gay men. *Journal of Addictive Diseases* 22 (4): 47-60.

Lenton, S., Boys, A., and Norcross, K. (1997). Raves, drugs and experience: Drug use by a sample of people who attend raves in Western Australia. *Addiction* 92 (10): 1327-1337.

Mansergh, G., Colfax, G. N., Marks, G., Rader, M., Guzman, R., and Buchbinder, S. (2001). The curcuit party men's health survey: Findings and implications for gay and bisexual men. *American Journal of Public Health* 91 (6): 953-958.

Mattison, A. M., Ross, M. W., Wolfson, T., and Franklin, D. (San Diego HIV Neurobehavioral Research Center Group) (2001). Circuit party attendance, club drug use, and unsafe sex in gay men. *Journal of Substance Abuse* 13 (1-2): 119-126.

McElrath, K., and McEvoy, K. (2002). Negative experiences on ecstasy: The role of drug, set and setting. *Journal of Psychoactive Drugs* 34 (2): 199-208.

McElrath, K., and McEvoy, K. (2001). Fact, fiction, and function: Mythmaking and the social construction of ecstasy use. *Substance Use and Misuse* 36 (1-2): 1-22.

Nencini, P. (2002). Shaman and the rave party: Social pharmacology of ecstasy. *Substance Use and Misuse* 37 (8-10): 923-939.

Parker, H. J., Aldridge, J., and Measham, F. (1998). *Illegal leisure: The normalization of adolescent recreational drug use. Adolescence and Society Series.* London: Routledge.

Parrott, A. C. (2004). Is ecstasy MDMA? A review of the proportion of ecstasy tablets containing MDMA, their dosage levels, and the changing perceptions of purity. *Psychopharmacology* 173 (3-4): 234-241.

Parrott, A. C., Buchanan, T., Scholey, A. B., Heffernan, T., Ling, J., and Rodgers, J. (2002). Ecstasy/MDMA attributed problems reported by novice, moderate and heavy recreational users. *Human Psychopharmacology* 17 (6): 309-312.

Parrott, A. C., Sisk, E., and Turner, J. J. (2000). Psychobiological problems in heavy 'ecstasy' (MDMA) poly-drug users. *Drug and Alcohol Dependence* 60 (1): 105-110.

Reynolds, S. (1999). *Generation Ecstasy: Into the world of techno and rave culture.* New York: Routledge.

Rodgers, J. (2000). Cognitive performance amongst recreational users of "ecstasy." *Psychopharmacology* 151 (1): 19-24.

Ross, M. W., Mattison, A. M., and Franklin, D. R. (2003). Club drugs and sex on drugs are associated with different motivations for gay circuit party attendance in men. *Substance Use and Misuse* 38 (8): 1173-1183.

Schensul, J. J. (2001). *The diffusion of MDMA use among urban youth in Hartford, CT: Implications for drug and HIV prevention in club drug users and their networks.* Bethesda, MD: MDMA/Ecstasy Research: Advances, Challenges, Future Directions: A Scientific Conference, NIDA, July 19-20.

Schensul, J., and Burkholder, G. (in press). Vulnerability, social networks, sites and selling as predictors of drug use among urban African American and Puerto Rican emerging adults. *Journal of Drug Issues: Special Issue on Drug Use and Emerging Adulthood*, S. Martin and H. White (Eds.).

Singer, M. (in press). *Something Dangerous: Emergent and changing illicit drug use and community health.* Long Grove, IL: Waveland Press.

Singer, M., Clair, S., Schensul, J., Huebner, C., Eiserman, J., Pino, R., and Garcia, J. (in press). Dust in the wind: The growing use of embalming fluid among youth in Hartford, CT. *Substance Use and Misuse.*

Singer, M., Juvalis, J. A., and Weeks, M. (2000). High on illy: Studying an emergent drug problem in Hartford, CT. *Medical Anthropology* 18: 365-388.

Sterk, C. E., Elifson, K. W., Theall, K. P., Greene, K., and Boeri, M. W. (2003). Ecstasy: A new hype or a new epidemic–what a snapshot can tell us. *Alcohol and Drug Study Group Bulletin* 36 (1): 2-5.

Yacoubian, G. S., Jr. (2002). Assessing the temporal relationship between race and ecstasy use among high school seniors. *Journal of Drug Education* 32 (3): 213-225.

Yacoubian, G. S., Jr., Boyle, C., Harding, C. A., and Loftus, E. A. (2003). It's a rave new world: Estimating the prevalence and perceived harm of ecstasy and other drug use among club rave attendees. *Journal of Drug Education* 33 (2): 187-196.

Zemishlany, Z., Aizenberg, D., and Weizman, A. (2001). Subjective effects of MDMA ('Ecstasy') on human sexual function. *European Psychiatry: The Journal of the Association of European Psychiatrists* 16: 127-130.

The Diffusion of Ecstasy
Through Urban Youth Networks

Jean J. Schensul, PhD
Sarah Diamond, PhD
William Disch, PhD
Rey Bermudez
Julie Eiserman, MA

SUMMARY. Ecstasy is a drug commonly associated with all-night, or all-weekend electronic dance events known as raves. Upper- and middle-class clubs, gay bars and clubs, and party venues are other common pub-

---

Jean J. Schensul is Senior Scientist and Founding Director of the Institute for Community Research.

Sarah Diamond is Research Associate at the Institute for Community Research.

William Disch is Psychologist/Senior Research Analyst at the Institute for Community Research.

Rey Bermudez is Community Researcher at the Institute for Community Research.

Julie Eiserman is Associate Research Scientist at the Hispanic Health Council.

Address correspondence to: Jean J. Schensul, Institute for Community Research, 2 Hartford Square West, Suite 100, Hartford, CT 06106 (E-mail: jean.schensul@ icrweb.org).

The authors express appreciation to members of the field research team who contributed to the data that form the basis of this paper, including Jose Garcia, MSW, Cristina Huebner, MA, Gus Lopez, Lorie Broomhall, PhD, and to other members of the investigator team including coinvestigators Margaret Weeks, PhD, Merrill Singer, PhD, and data analyst, Gary Burkholder, PhD.

Research for this paper was supported by NIDA Grant #RFA DA-010101 (Urban Lifestyles: Club Drugs, Resource Inequities and Health Risks in Urban Youth) and NIDA Grant # R01-DA11421 (Pathways to High-Risk Drug Use Among Urban Youth).

[Haworth co-indexing entry note]: "The Diffusion of Ecstasy Through Urban Youth Networks." Schensul, Jean J. et al. Co-published simultaneously in *Journal of Ethnicity in Substance Abuse* (The Haworth Press, Inc.) Vol. 4, No. 2, 2005, pp. 39-71; and: *New Drugs on the Street: Changing Inner City Patterns of Illicit Consumption* (ed: Merrill Singer) The Haworth Press, Inc., 2005, pp. 39-71. Single or multiple copies of this article are available for a fee from The Haworth Document Delivery Service [1-800-HAWORTH, 9:00 a.m. - 5:00 p.m. (EST). E-mail address: docdelivery@haworthpress.com].

lic settings where ecstasy use occurs. During the mid to late 1990s its use was reported in locations as distant as Australia and New Zealand, England and Scotland, and North America. In the United States, use increased dramatically at the end of the millennium, and drug monitoring systems began to report its presence among urban youth. Using social influence, social marketing and diffusion theory, this paper outlines the micro-level processes through which ecstasy traveled from downtown clubs catering to suburban young adults through urban youth networks through distributors and users. The paper is based on participant observation, and in-depth interviews with dealers and users collected during the period of peak diffusion 1999-2001, and survey data collected from 401 poly-drug users between the ages of 16 and 24 and collected at two time points from 1999-2002. *[Article copies available for a fee from The Haworth Document Delivery Service: 1-800-HAWORTH. E-mail address: <docdelivery@haworthpress.com> Website: <http://www.HaworthPress.com> © 2005 by The Haworth Press, Inc. All rights reserved.]*

KEYWORDS. Ecstasy, inner city youth, African American, Latino, drug selling

INTRODUCTION

MDMA (3,4-methylenedioxymethanphetamine) is widely known in the United States and globally as a dance drug associated with raves, parties, and other nighttime recreational functions (Fitzgerald & Hamilton, 1994; Forsyth, 1996; Forsyth, Barnard, & McKeganey, 1997; Lewis & Ross, 1995; Merchant & Macdonald, 1994; Riley & Hayward, 2004; Solowij, Hall, & Lee, 1992). Most users reported in the literature are working-class or professional youth and young adults including gay men, who take it to enhance their recreational experiences in bar, club or dance settings (Hunt & Evans, 2003; Lee, Galanter, Dermatis, & McDowell, 2003; Mattison, Ross, Wolfson, Franklin, & San Diego, 2001; Romanelli, Smith, & Pomeroy, 2003; Ross, Mattison, & Franklin, 2003; Tong & Boyer, 2002). Recent research has suggested that its availability and use has spread beyond the downtown and underground rave "scene" and has extended into urban African American, West Indian, Latino and other ethnic minority networks (Yacoubian, 2002a; Yacoubian, Jr., 2003; Yacoubian, Arria, Fost, & Wish, 2002; Yacoubian, Boyle, Harding, & Loftus, 2003).

Ecstasy, like other popular drugs, is a global commodity (Agar & Reisinger, 2003; Hunt & Evans, 2003), marketed in association with a hegemonic consumer lifestyle that includes an emphasis on social status and group membership acquired through commodities or material goods (music, clothing, jewelry, etc.), access to socially desirable sites and settings, and pleasure (recreational activities, sensual experiences, dancing). Diffusion has been noted across continents, marketed through music, travel and tourism, and entrepreneurial activity (Calafat et al., 2001; Calafat & Stocco, 2000). But the micro-level processes through which club drugs diffuse across settings/venues and classes and into the general population have not been accounted for in the literature. This paper focuses on microlevel processes of distribution and use that illustrate the ways in which a new multi-purpose club drug, ecstasy, moved from the club, rave, and bar settings where it was first available in association with dance events, to urban neighborhoods and youth networks, generating a new consumer market. It is based on data collected in a small eastern industrial city during the period from 1999-2001 when reported ecstasy use was peaking nationally (Wallace et al., 2002; Yacoubian, 2003). A team of researchers in Hartford, CT, were able to observe the diffusion of ecstasy from suburban users and downtown clubs into urban groups of users through networks of distributors, and to document both the expansion of use and availability (Eiserman, Singer, Schensul, & Broomhall, 2003; Schensul, 2001). The paper will apply diffusion and social influence theories to the ways in which MDMA was introduced, accepted and normalized as an important element in the drug repertoire of urban youth.

History of Ecstasy

Ecstasy represents an innovation in drug use. It first appeared in recreational drug use during the mid-80s. Its use was promoted in northern Europe by tourists and entrepreneurs returning from southern Europe (Spain and other areas of the Mediterranean) where all-night party culture was an indigenous cultural phenomenon, and ecstasy supported disinhibition and provided the fuel to sustain all-night dancing to techno and house music (Bellis, Hughes, Bennett, & Thomson, 2003; Elliott et al., 1998). By the mid-90s ecstasy was widely used in England, Australia, resort islands and large cities of the U.S. with a significant all-night club life, including New York and San Francisco (Forsyth, 1996; Lenton, Boys, & Norcross, 1997; Weir, 2000). By the late 1990s, it began to diffuse to suburban and rural areas, and into urban neighborhoods of the United States (Yacoubian et al., 2002). Rural users were introduced to it through clandestine raves–large private electronic dance events that mimicked the electronic music club and after-hours scene in large urban centers. In the United States, as in England and Scotland, these events were marked by significant drug use, not dissimilar to the widespread drug use typical of music concerts and other popular cultural events in the 1970s (Parker, Aldridge, & Measham, 1998; Tong & Boyer, 2002). Ecstasy and (to a much lesser extent) other so-called designer or club drugs combined with alcohol, marijuana, cocaine, and in gay club circles methamphetamine, were the drugs of choice in these party settings (Brecht & von Mayrhauser, 2002; Colfax et al., 2001).

American national drug monitoring systems identified the presence and increasing use of ecstasy during the latter half of the 1990s (Maxwell, 2003, 2004). These sources of information did not show ecstasy as a drug of choice among African American or Latino youth. Instead, use seemed to be concentrated among suburban white high school and college students (Yacoubian, 2002b). By 1999, our research in Hartford, Connecticut uncovered the presence of ecstasy in the context of a study of transitions to hard drug use in urban African American and Latino adolescents and young adults. While recruiting study participants in the clubs and after-hours in the city, ethnographers identified ecstasy as a new drug, and encountered young Latinos who had tried it, and were obtaining or purchasing it in club settings from other youth or house dealers. This transferring of drug norms, strategies for obtaining ecstasy, and information about use from suburban/college users to urban users reversed the standard stereotypes about the city as the primary source of drugs for suburban drug users. It also raised our concern over the possibility that young Latinos might be harassed or charged with ecstasy or other drug-dealing by watchful bouncers and police officers monitoring these sites. This concern was heightened with the introduction of the harsh sentencing guidelines for dealing ecstasy which were established through The Illicit Drug Anti-Proliferation Act of 2003 (S.226), formerly known as the "Rave Act." Another major concern was that new urban users might know little about the drug except for its perceived effect, and might not take proper precautions to protect themselves from the effects of mixing with other drugs, dehydration, overhydration, adulteration and midweek depression. Further, we did not know whether ecstasy, despite being heavily marketed through the media and by rappers, would become popular with urban youth (Diamond et al., 2004). Thus we mounted a substudy to monitor the process of diffusion of X into the urban environment, patterns of use, the ways it might become integrated into urban youth drug repertoires and how youth were coping with its use.

SOCIAL NORMS, SOCIAL INFLUENCE, AND THE DIFFUSION OF NEW DRUGS

Social norms theory emphasizes the formation and presence of expectations and standards for behavior in the social environment, including socially acceptable patterns of drug use. Norms are formed through interpersonal relationships that reinforce beliefs and behaviors, enhance competence and encourage persistence (Guisinger & Blatt, 1994; Harter, 1990a, 1990b). These processes of interpersonal exchange underlie constructivist approaches to knowledge generation and group norms (Berger & Luckmann, 1966; Rogoff, 2003; Vygotsky, 1978; Wertsch, 1991), which in turn contribute to the development of individual cognitions and behavior and to the evolution and transmission of culture (e.g., Bearison, 1982; Guisinger & Blatt, 1994). Generally, this approach is used to frame intervention theory designed to promote positive social norms or to modify social norms present among peers, through communication and role modeling (Donaldson, Graham, & Hansen, 1994: 212). But it can also be utilized to illustrate how youth are persuaded to experiment with and sustain use of new drugs, especially those drugs such as marijuana, alcohol, and ecstasy that are believed to enhance the quality of social interaction.

The role of social influence in sustaining existing social norms and initiating new ones has been documented theoretically and through application in interventions (Hawkins, Hill, Guo, & Battin-Pearson, 2002; Latkin, 1995; Maxwell, 2002; Sale, 1999). In the diffusion of innovations, social influence occurs through the degree of correspondence or similarity (*homophily*) of those modeling the innovation (the agents) with members of the target population and the target population's degree of acceptance (trust) of agents (Friedman, DesJarlais, & Ward, 1994; Latané, Liu, Nowak, Bonevento, & Zheng, 1995; Latané, 1995; Newmeyer, Feldman, Biernacki, & Watters, 1989; Nowak, Szamrej, & Latané, 1990). Rogers and others note that these are important characteristics in influencing the individual's decision to accept new behaviors or technology. Dynamic Social Impact Theory (DSIT) adds to the understanding of social influence through communication, three central characteristics which increase likelihood of acceptance of new ideas (new drugs): *strength*, or the relative *power* people (face-to-face or through the media) have to influence others (through similarity or homophily or other characteristics, such as wealth, or social status); *immediacy*, defined as the physical or social space between influencing agents and those being influenced; and *number* of people communicating the new message to the individual (Latané et al., 1995; Latané, Nowak, & Liu, 1994; Nowak et al., 1990). This perspective is consistent with constructuralist approaches to communications in which repeated multiple simultaneous acts of communication between agents in a social setting change relationships, concepts, norms, and the setting itself (Kaufer & Carley, 1993).

Social marketing aims to sell commodities by utilizing principles of social influence such as those specified in the DSIT model above. Social marketing of a new drug utilizes the same components as a social marketing approach to change social norms. Both are intended to change individual behavior at the group or aggregate level (Black, Blue, & Coster, 2001). Social marketing of ecstasy requires delivery of materials, messages and processes that appeal to core values and promise tangible benefits while minimizing risks associated with use. *Promotion* involves incentives and other means that improve awareness of the drug and the need for its use. *Price* refers to social, psychological, financial and other human resource costs of using ecstasy, and *place* refers to distribution channels for delivering the product (venues and persons). Social marketing segments the market, developing specific messages and formats appealing to specific subgroups or niches within a larger market or audience (Flocks et al., 2001). Social norms, social influence, and social marketing provide a systematic framework for understanding how distributors made use of local culture, context and market to promote the use of a new drug, ecstasy, and participate in its diffusion.

STUDY SETTING

Data for this paper were collected through a NIDA funded study,[1] a collaboration of the Institute for Community Research and the Hispanic Health Council, conducted during the period 1998-2002 in Hartford, Connecticut, a mid-sized city of approximately 130,000 in the northeastern United States. Hartford is known as one of the poorest cities in the country, with a depressed economy, high school dropout rate and limited opportunities for urban youth and young adults to find sustainable employment in the country. In terms of ethnic composition, approximately 45% of the city's population is Latino (mainly Puerto

Rican, with increasing numbers of South Americans, Dominicans, Mexicans and Central Americans), 35% African American, and 10% West Indian Caribbean. Other residents include working class white ethnic groups (Italian, Irish, and French), single professionals working in insurance, financing, health and post-secondary education, and new immigrants from central Europe (Poland and Bosnia) and Southeast Asia who are developing an economic base through small business development.

Hartford has been undergoing a slow process of gentrification sponsored and managed by the city and state governments in partnership with public and private development ventures. Consequences of this process have been the destruction of family-based public housing projects, with subsequent decentralization of families to low-cost rental areas in the city or surrounding municipalities, and residential and recreational development in and bordering on the city's downtown area. Developments include an expansion of upscale downtown nightlife, and the construction of a major recreational area (sports and conference arena, shopping mall and high-cost condominiums and residential apartment buildings) along the Connecticut River.

Hartford is located along the main transportation route between New York and Springfield, Massachusetts, and is only 90 minutes from the Boston area. Young people in what could be termed the "New England Party Culture Region" move along the major highways (95 and 91 North-South and 84 East-West) obtaining a variety of drugs used for recreational purposes at different venues and taking advantage of new party opportunities at clubs, bars, all-ages sites and other locations in the major urban areas along Interstate Highway 91 (Bridgeport, New Haven, Hartford and Springfield). Clubs advertise openings, special nights, performances, and drink specials through fliers, cards, and word of mouth, as well as on the Internet, to attract young people from across the Northeastern seaboard. The Hartford region alone includes a number of large hotels, five major universities with thousands of undergraduate and graduate level students, and more than 65 clubs and bars popular among youths across classes and ethnicities, making it a major location for nighttime party life and associated drug use.

For this paper we draw on qualitative data gathered through participant observation and informal and formal in-depth interviews with drug distributors, drug users, and youths attending a variety of recreational events over the period from 1998-2002. Some of the data were collected with support from the parent study and some through a supplement funded to the parent grant through the Office of AIDS Research to study ecstasy use and HIV. The Institutional Review Board of the Institute for Community Research approved the study and its supplements each year.

METHODS

Ethnographic Data

Two Puerto Rican and two Anglo-American ethnographers collected ethnographic data on youth poly-drug-using social networks and ecstasy use. Ethnographers conducted regular observations in community settings and downtown clubs and bars during a two-year period, 1999-2001. Through street ethnography, one of the ethnographers identified networks of youths who were involved in using and trading drugs both in the community and in several downtown clubs. She was able to follow these networks, revealing how they obtained, used and traded ecstasy with their friends and what accounted for their effectiveness in shifting their business toward the sale of a new drug.

At the same time, site observations identified and documented ecstasy and other drug-selling, using and purchasing rules, practices, and infrastructure in a number of different recreational locations. In-depth interviews with ecstasy users, some of whom were also lower level distributors, provided information about how users used, shared and described the drug to their friends and about how ecstasy was marketed to local users. All respondents who completed in-depth interviews signed a consent form and were paid $25.00 on completion of the interview. Interviews were transcribed, entered into Atlas Ti, a text management program, coded by one researcher and checked by a second for reliability.

Survey data (N = 401) were collected at two time-points 15 months apart beginning in the fall of 1999. Participants were recruited using a targeted sampling plan in selected neighborhoods of the city (Singer & Weeks, 1992; Watters & Biernacki, 1989). Eligibility for enrollment included 30-day use of alcohol or marijuana (regular or high THC) and at least one other non-injected drug. A supplement to the survey was added midway that asked about club drugs and participation in party life. Participants received $25.00 for each survey completed (baseline, 15-month follow-up, and Club Supplement). The survey included demographic, family, peer, school and work risk and protective factors, current and past drug use, and questions related to drug selling, violence exposure, and sexual risk. This paper draws on data from the baseline survey and club supplement (N = 206).

MARKETING ECSTASY:
DOWNTOWN "CLUBS" AND "AFTER-HOURS"

In the late 1990s, downtown Hartford's nightlife offered a meeting ground for young adults between the ages of 15 and 30. Socialization options included "regular" clubs (open until 2 AM and serving alcohol), "after-hours" clubs (open after 2 AM and serving sodas, water and a dance environment) and various bars, and restaurants. Some clubs and "after-hours" were under the same ownership, and young patrons were encouraged to go to both sites, depending on the time of night. At the start of our study, in 1998-9, most of the downtown sites catered to Caucasian youth, mainly older high school and college students and young professionals with electronic techno music and a rave-like environment. Gradually, Latino and some African American youth began to attend some of the clubs and after-hours, especially those that featured special nights or "floors" dedicated to Latin, Hip Hop or Reggae music. Halls and other large spaces in the northern part of the city were locations for irregularly scheduled rave-like events that drew youth from the suburbs and attracted African American breakdancers (B-boys) from the city to perform and compete. These locations and special events created specific occasions or opportunity structures where urban, suburban and college youth crossed paths, socialized, partied together and traded drugs.

A number of researchers have described the commercial and symbolic importance of drug and alcohol use in club settings (Boyd, McCabe, & d'Arcy, 2003; Breslau, 2002). Some drugs associated with "date rape" (e.g., Ketamine, GHB and Rohypnol) were known to be dangerous, especially when mixed with alcohol, and had limited distribution, especially in New England (J. Maxwell, 2004). Other drugs, most notably ecstasy, were viewed as offering benefits to late night recreation including the enhancement of sensation, sociability, energy sustainability and sexuality. Many, though not all, participants reported learning about ecstasy for the first time in association with club and after-hour environments, and described buying, selling and using ecstasy in these sites.

Buying and Selling Ecstasy in Club Environments

Drugs and alcohol are viewed as part of weekend (Thursday through Sunday) nighttime "chillin'" or "partying," and locations are known because they offer alcohol specials and markets for specific drugs (for example, cocaine), specialized or higher quality versions of specific drugs (for example, strong or flavored "dust" or PCP) or drugs in general. In response to the rave trend which was sweeping across America, a number of clubs deliberately tried to create rave-like environments, featuring techno music, light shows and products catering to dancers. Water bottles, back packs, lollipops, pacifiers and glowsticks, all products associated with ecstasy use, were also sold in some locations. Vicks Vaporub, masks and other materials to enhance the effects of the ecstasy were not sold, but their use was not prohibited. Local clubs either ignored or were uninformed about the association of these products with MDMA use. A photograph of a local dance event in a warehouse in the city's north end in 2000-1, showed youths dancing with glowsticks and using masks with a caption praising the site for its safe environment. In 2001, an ecstasy dealer was arrested for being the "house dealer" at one of the downtown clubs. The dealer reported that the club was fully aware of his activities, and the owners were compensated weekly with a sum of $1000, for allowing the dealer exclusive access to sell in that location.

Depending on the location, drugs may be sold only by house dealers or by both house dealers and dealers who come to participate in the scene and to distribute their products. Establishments may not be directly involved in the sale of illegal substances but their financial success depends on their ability to attract youth who favor alcohol, dance music, the availability of drugs and/or the ability to use them in or around the premises. There is the perception, as summarized by several respondents, that club owners are involved in bulk purchase and distribution of ecstasy and other drugs, and that money from the sale of drugs helps to support the operation of the location.[2]

> The one that was really running that place, it was, it used to be you know what I'm saying, mafia niggas. You never seen mafia niggas driving real new, real sharp cars that's the mafia niggas ok them niggas. All right, one time my brother came inside boom. My brother was anyway a'ight, he was getting rid of it, then they took my brother inside a room, I mean they showed sandwich bags, sandwich bags full of hot to the top ecstasy—who's selling it—the

own club–how else do you think those club be making enough money to pay everyone else?

A second participant noted that in one club they don't ask for identification and people sell drugs there. In response to the interviewer's question as to whether the club knows about that, the respondent said: "I think they do cause you're not gonna tell me that on the dance floor people smoking marihuana, place full of smoke, you understand, one bathroom for men and women, one bathroom only, understand? It's something that's super logical that the guy knows."

In the city, the most popular party drugs have been alcohol, marijuana and cocaine. Other drugs are available, but urban youth normally have not used them. Between 1999 and 2001, key informants and observations pointed to ecstasy as a new "social" drug (as defined by preference for use in association with other people rather than alone). Ecstasy was first described in several of Hartford's downtown clubs.

> P. The last time I went was about a month ago . . . And I tell you this place is, you know, it's for people that are drugged up, high. You see the women on the dance floor touching themselves all over, real horny. You see the men . . ., that's something you go to the bathroom and you see people using drugs in the bathroom. And for real the place, I don't know how that place is still open.
> I. What drugs do the people there use?
> P. Heroin, cocaine, marihuana, ecstasy . . . everything, alcohol. . . .

Another participant said:

> If the bouncers know that you're selling ecstasy, they won't let you in. They won't let you in because they feel like you stepping on their turf. Cause that's their turf. So, like if you're an outsider, like if I wanted to go in there, and be like, you know I got pills to sell, if the bouncers found out, they'll kick you in half a minute, they'll bounce you out. Like a lot of people go to the club cause they know they can find the drugs safely in there. They don't have to go to the block and you know, get caught buying it. . . . that's the main reason why a lot of kids go there. Cause they can find it there and you don't have to be like watching over your shoulder to have the cops coming.

This same interviewee reported being invited with friends and husband into the club's VIP room. The youth who invited them emerged with marijuana and ecstasy from the VIP room (a private room or floor with a separate entrance fee and monitored entrance, where drugs may be sold and sex sometimes takes place). According to the interviewee "whatever you wanted, they was in that room . . ." The interviewee said:

> never been in that room because we usually when we go we're usually already on the pill, we don't go buy the pills in there. But we know people that have been in that room, and that's where they get it from. I mean we heard, there's a friend of ours that goes there, like every weekend and the weekend that he doesn't miss. The bouncer already knows him, he, he just lets him in, he'll be like all right, go right in and . . . then he goes to the bar. He knows everybody in the bar, like if they really, really like, like you, and you don't cause them any trouble, you don't make trouble, you don't, you know, do anything you just sit there and do whatever you do there, they really like that . . . 'cause they know that you know, we can trust this person, we can trust him, you know, he's okay.

Another respondent reported that (he) only sold ecstasy in a club. When the interviewer asked how someone would ask for some, he said:

> 'cause people are stupid and they would ask for it. They would walk up and say "Yo, you got 'E'? Do you know who got the 'E'? Can you find me some?" Well I can find you some "E," but it is going to cost you some. We are in the club. It is late night. I don't know if you are undercover, I'm taking a risk. They would be willing to accept my stories and they would be willing to pay.

Summing it up, a young man emphasized: "'cause that's what the club is like built on. Like the club is open market for ecstasy. To everybody."

Survey Data on Use of Ecstasy in Clubs

Survey data were collected in 2000-2001 from a subsample of 206 people in the parent study who responded to a supplement asking about club drugs and club related activities. This group of 206 young male and female African American and Latino participants in the parent study confirmed that ecstasy ranked high as a drug of choice associated with club, and other party activities. Among more than 12 drugs listed, only ecstasy use (ever) is associated with attending a Hartford club (χ^2 = 11.636; Df = 1; Sig. = .001).

The subsample was asked whether they had ever used, bought or sold in a club each one of a list of drugs that urban youth typically use (see Table 1). Most respondents had used alcohol, and regular and exotic marijuana in a club. Slightly less than half had used ecstasy and "dust" or PCP, and much fewer numbers had used other drugs. About half had purchased marijuana and ecstasy in clubs. Fewer had purchased alcohol or "dust." Alcohol is expensive, many participants were underage and some of the clubs they referred to were all-ages or after-hours clubs where alcohol was not served though drugs were available on the premises.

These respondents reported almost no use of those drugs typically referred to as "club drugs"–rohypnol, GHB, methamphetamine and Ketamine. Much lower percentages of youth reported selling drugs in a club, a risky activity at best. Contrary to common stereotypes about patterns of drug selling by urban youth to suburban users, participants in our study reported selling marijuana but not heroin or any form of cocaine in these settings. Ethnicity was an important factor only with reference to ecstasy use and purchase. At the time of the study, Puerto Rican youth were more likely to have used and bought ecstasy in a club than African Americans, but not to have sold it. Other survey data confirm that Puerto Rican youth were more involved in both using and selling ecstasy in other settings. There were no other differences across ethnic groups with respect to using, buying and selling club drugs.

TABLE 1. Drugs Used, Bought and Sold in Clubs (N = 401)

	Used in Club	Bought in Club	Sold in Club
Alcohol	93%	30%	4%
Regular marijuana	80%	54%	36%
Exotic marijuana	74%	51%	28%
Ecstasy	45%	45%	13%
Dust (marijuana with embalming fluid)	46%	23%	10%
Hallucinogens	11%	20%	1%
Special K	4%	9%	1%
Crystal Meth.	1%	0%	1.5%

Diffusion of X into Hartford's Neighborhoods

Newspaper and other accounts reflect attention paid to ecstasy use during the period from 2000-2002. These reports mention the arrest of student ecstasy dealers on the University of Connecticut campus or suburban area (November 20, 1999; January 10, 2000; April 4, 2000; May 14, 2000), deaths of college and suburban high school students from consuming alcohol and ecstasy (2000 and 2002), and arrests of suburban high school students for using ecstasy (November 22, 2000). In January 2001, three clubs, two of which were owned by the same owner, were shut down by the DEA and local police because of the presence and use of ecstasy and other drugs on the premises. These clubs re-opened shortly thereafter (January 23, 2001) under police observation, and with videotaping and patting down of patrons. During this time, some arrests of street dealers for selling ecstasy took place (January 23, 2000). In 2000-01, a teen was arrested in Hartford for selling ecstasy in downtown bars (October 4, 2000), another teen for selling on the street (January 2, 2001) and another for manufacturing ecstasy at home (April 13, 2001). Those arrested in all of these instances were young adults, between the ages of 16 and 24. These reports reflected the first steps in the expansion of ecstasy from suburban to urban club and street markets.

Our ethnographic data on drug dealing provide us with an early example of a drug distribution network that introduced ecstasy to Hartford's neighborhoods. This cross-neighborhood drug dealing enterprise network successfully managed to establish a marijuana distribution business by working through four discrete personal networks of trusted drug dealers built over more than a decade in different neighborhoods of the city. The head of this network was a young entrepreneur, connected to bulk marijuana and cocaine distributors. Although he chose to avoid selling cocaine because he perceived it to be too dangerous, he was able to use his cocaine connections to obtain ecstasy, which he then sold through established marijuana distribution networks. Following is the story of this young entrepreneur's success and eventual decline.

Franky is a young (approximately 30 years of age) Puerto Rican male. He grew up in the Puerto Rican community of Hartford and his family is well-known in the community. His father, a former mid-level drug dealer, had been employed in a social service career at the time of the study. His family had connections to large-scale drug distributors several of whom were family members themselves, and who offered him opportunities from time to time that he found difficult to resist.

Franky is a charismatic young man who completed high school and found a full-time position working in the criminal justice system and a part-time position in a public sector educational resource. These jobs provided him with economic security, and the safety of settings in which he could meet, establish and maintain links with potential future drug users and dealers and meet with them in public without fear of observation or discovery.

Franky learned about ecstasy while attending a downtown club. He tried it, liked it, and purchased some to share with his "boys" outside of the club setting. He had a large and diffuse network of friends who were also dealers that he had carefully built over a decade or more. While in his teen years, his family moved from one neighborhood to another across the city, first in the city's mainly African American North End, and then in various locations in the Primarily Latino south end. With his social skills he was able to make close friends in each of the neighborhoods and across ethnic and age boundaries. A natural leader, he was able to establish his own clique in every neighborhood and to maintain its independence in the face of competition from other groups, including national gangs who were recruiting from local crews in the mid-1990s. When Franky's family moved to another neighborhood, he maintained contact with his group, and in this way was able to develop and sustain close personal relationships with people in areas of the city that varied in ethnicity and at times competed with one another. By the time he became one of the study's key informants, anxious to tell his story, he was managing five separate marijuana selling networks. He obtained high-quality marijuana from a distributor whom he referred to as "Hero," and then redistributed it for sale to his networks. Network members were trusted in their neighborhoods, had their long-term contacts and clients, took their percentage and returned profits to Franky.

When "Hero" went to jail, he asked Franky to take over his business. Franky agreed to do this but only for several years, until he was able to make enough money to leave drug-selling behind. When "Hero" approached him with the idea of selling ecstasy, Franky had already tried it, liked it, and shared it with his teams. He saw the potential value of the market and was prepared to add ecstasy to his repertoire. He began to distribute it through his networks across the city. His network members were trusted members of their communities, similar in age and ethnicity to clients. They were users who could share their experiences, were known to sell quality products, and who could act as role models and opinion leaders for potential clients in their own communities. Franky's ability to bridge across small ethnic and neighborhood-specific networks of user/distributors, placed him in a significant position to be able to promote and disseminate new products rapidly, efficiently and safely across the entire city.

Undoubtedly there were other distributors like Franky who, over time, created a local street market for ecstasy. The following year, our research team was able to identify several sites, one in the north part of Hartford, and a second in the southern part of the city near an urban college campus that constituted central locations for purchasing ecstasy. Subsequently, as the urban market group, dealers began to sell ecstasy as part of their drug repertoire in various locations throughout the city. In the next example, one of many, a respondent describes how he obtains pills, sells them on the street to everyone, mainly people he knows, takes a cut and returns the money to the supplier.

> P. he just gave me ten (pills). . . . when I be done I'll come back with all that money.
> I. and how much he will give it to you, how much money he would give to you? Out of it you sell ten pills, how much money would you get?
> P. I get three dollars out of each pill.
> I. and they go quick or do they take time?
> P. fast.
> I. you said that usually in the streets, in clubs or?
> P. in the streets . . . For twenty dollars.
> I. twenty; do you sell it to everybody, do you sell it to friends?
> P. I sell it to everybody . . . some girl friends, girls that go to the clubs. They be like, yo you got the "e"? they ask for it.
> I. so usually they are friends of yours?
> P. yea, sometimes, sometimes people come that I don't know and sometimes I don't sell it.

This respondent purchased ecstasy from Latino dealers who sold it outside their neighborhood.

> I. Do you know if they sell that in the North End?
> R. They sell it too.
> I. More in the south.
> C. More over here (south end).
> I. So the Latin sells it more?
> C. Yeah.

Another respondent said that though ecstasy was more easily found in other larger cities, like Philadelphia, it could be found in Hartford. "Here's what, here if you want them, you usually got to go . . . ecstasy you either gotta go, there's a place in the North End that, down Sherwood Avenue that sells ecstasy . . . Simpson Circle . . . sells ecstasy." However, he noted that it was easier to obtain them at the clubs: "If you find 'em out here, you're lucky." Most respondents agreed that it was much easier to find ecstasy in the city and to buy it from street dealers in 2000 than it had been in the past. Toward the end of the study period, respondents were noting that ecstasy was widely available all over Hartford, on the streets, through known contacts, and in local clubs.

> The whole Hartford sell ecstasy now. It's not. . . . Like before, when it first came out it was so hard to get a pill and . . . wherever they sell weed they sell E Pills.

> It's not at the same level as heroin or dope, I mean marijuana, but it has gone up. Because I'm telling you about three years ago I knew about ecstasy but it was hard to get it and nowadays you can go anywhere and you can get it fast.

Currently field researchers note that street or electronic drug dealers maintain a repertoire of preferred drugs that include ecstasy, but do not specialize in ecstasy because the market is intermittent (mainly weekends rather than daily) even among regular club or party goers.

WAYS OF DISTRIBUTING AND OBTAINING ECSTASY

Ecstasy is distributed and obtained in a number of different ways. Homophily, trust, social proximity and social influence all play a significant role in the diffusion, marketing, selling and use of ecstasy. The typical ways of procuring ecstasy are by getting it free from close friends, pooling money so that friends can purchase and distribute small amounts from their dealers, or purchasing it directly from friends who sell it in smaller or larger amounts. It can also be purchased from identified local distributors in clubs or parties. There have been continuing reports that ecstasy is distributed free of charge in private hotel parties that link urban and suburban youth, as a disinhibitor to set the stage for creative sexual experimentation, or in home settings that cater to initiates and younger users.

Getting It Free from Friends

The retail or street price of ecstasy has remained at $20.00-$25.00 per pill over the past four years although occasionally respondents report that they can negotiate cheaper prices. With costs prohibitive, one way to provide an incentive for the use of ecstasy especially to new users is for trusted friends to make them available free of charge. Our field notes reflect many reports from users who obtained their first pill from friends free of charge. Providing ecstasy free of charge is a typical way to market a new drug product, while at the same time enhancing prestige and status (Schensul et al., 2000). Users may persuade their friends to use ecstasy despite intentions to avoid it. Those who enjoy it will try to use it again, but more than likely, they will have to pay for it.

> P. The pill, my friend gave it to me.
> I. But did she buy it in the club or did she . . .
> P. Uh Uh. She been had them already. I was in the car when she got it. But I ain't see who it was. She just went out of the car and said "I'll be back" or whatever, and then she came back like "Oh I got some pills!" I was like, "I ain't trying no pills," but I ended up trying it. . . . she got it on, I think, South Mansfield on North End–I think South Mansfield on the Sound End right (this street [pseudonym] is mid-town bordering on northern and southern neighborhoods of Hartford which probably explains why this respondent was confused about the location).

Another respondent also said that his friend had purchased ecstasy for about $25.00 and gave him one.

> P. And the friend that gave it to you, did you buy it off him or did he just give it to you?
> I. He bought it off of one of his friends. He paid something like $25.00.

A third described how he convinced one of his friends to try it.

> Yeah, so it was around my 18th birthday. I asked my best friend to try it. He was like, "No, I don't wanna try it. I don't wanna try it." He's like, "I'll go anyway and have a good time." Everybody else was trying it. Or did it. Or has done it. Or whatever. So we're in the line and he's like, "You know what? Screw it! Just give it to me." I

gave it to him. I felt kinda bad because, well, I didn't really peer pressure him, but everyone else was doing it. He probably felt outta place. "Hey man, c'mon, just one time, you just try it. You don't like it, y'know, don't do it again . . . ever." So he tried it . . . we're in a long line and had to wait. "I'm not gonna have a good time. I'm not gonna have a good time." Next thing you know, he gets inside and you can't get the kid off the dance floor. We wanna leave and this kid is f**** going at it, like . . . I mean, hopping around and I mean, this dude was just out of it. He didn't wanna leave. To make a long story short, he ended up liking it, and did it a few times after, then more . . . like I said, more of my friends starting getting into it.

Purchasing It from Friends

Most friends, however, are less generous with their drug supply. Survey respondents, including first-time users, generally purchase pills from their friends who are dealers and who they trust.

> I. I want to go back to the first time that you did it. Did you guys pay for it or did someone buy it for you . . .
> P. Um, we had to pay for it. We had got it from one of our friends, he had, I guess he had started selling it. And then . . .
> I. Is he Puerto Rican?
> P. Yeah, Yeah, he's Puerto Rican. And we got it from him . . . it was about $20.00 a pill.

Another respondent said that her friend gets it from people she knows,

> people that sell 'em or, old friends she know. . . . Or if not, she goes–she used to go to (club), and go inside there. She used to spend like two hundred dollars and she used to get twelve for two hundred.

This exemplifies a typical pattern in which users and small-scale suppliers bargain for cheaper bulk prices, usually from 10 to 20 pills. They can bargain more effectively if the suppliers are their friends. Bulk purchases may be on behalf of friends, to sell to friends, or to sell to others they know as well as to use themselves. Bulk price reductions are incentives both to buy and sell ecstasy. Friends who are dealers will sometimes reduce the price of ecstasy for their friends. One participant said in her experience, the cheapest price for ecstasy was $10.00 and that she got it for that price only because "that's my boy. That is the only reason I got it for that cheap, but he still charged me . . . everybody else, it was either twenty or twenty-five." Regular users know the typical cost of a pill (ranging from $20-$25) and will turn down an opportunity to purchase them for more, especially if the dealer is a stranger.

Selling to friends or even to anonymous buyers sometimes involves requesting feedback about the quality of the drug or the experience while high, especially if the dealer is promoting ecstasy over other drugs. One dealer who encouraged clients to use ecstasy said:

> P. I'd tell them to come back and tell me, and they used to come back and tell me that they liked the way that they felt, and that they–it was like 'cause I don't know, and they said that they felt like they still had dope in their system cause, I don't know, to me, that pill has cocaine, dope, all that other stuff, whatever it has . . . .
> I. So what was their response?
> P. They said they liked ecstasy, yes.

He is able to use the quotes he receives from his clients to promote the quality of his product.

Sometimes purchasing through personal networks includes direct social persuasion. For example, this same participant said that he told a woman who used to buy dope from him to try ecstasy.

> then I told her to try ecstasy or whatever, and I brought her the pill. She gave me the money and I brought her the pill and she didn't used to come buy dope off of me no more, she used to come buy ecstasy . . . she stopped using dope to use ecstasy . . . to me, I think ecstasy is better than any drug.

In a form of indirect influence, another respondent said that she had used it first with family and friends at a friend's house in preparation for going to an after-hours in a community outside of Hartford. Her friend, a user and a seller, introduced ecstasy to her, and then sold it to her which she found quite acceptable:

> In the drug world, nothing's, nothing is free. It is true, nothing in life is free, nothing. Unless you're the one who supplies it. Then it's free to you. Other than that, it's not free, just how it goes I guess.

Subsequently, she reported, she purchased ecstasy from known people around the neighborhood. She said that personal relationships were important when buying ecstasy, and that further, as a quality check, they observed others including the dealer while using the drugs (modeling the effects) before they used them, to make sure the drugs were safe.

> Everywhere else we went (besides one specific club) we knew somebody who had it. If it wasn't our boy, it was a boy of a boy that we knew. We always knew somebody, like we had chilled with them, and we've, we've seen them on "E" before we've taken it. That's just how we are; we are very conscientious people. We would rather see somebody else take it and see how it affects them before we put it in our body. . . . it worked because it was like this. If we seen that person taking it and he had a bad high, then we wouldn't take it because they we knew, all right, then there is something funny about it. But if he took it and he just enjoyed the high with us, we would be like all right then, we should have to take it. (The person who took it) was either the person we bought it from or somebody that was real close to us that just didn't care and would try anything.

Purchasing can be done face-to-face as described above, or electronically. Purchasing ecstasy and other drugs electronically is increasingly the norm because of its safety for both the seller and the buyer. One respondent who purchased ecstasy on the street described how she would obtain a pill late in the evening.

> I. If you wanted a pill and it was nine o'clock, how would you get one?
> P. I still have their phone numbers. I would just call them, or if somebody . . . already who was on their way to get one and I just gave them my money and they would get me one. . . . we always had to go to them.
> I. Where would you normally go, to their houses?
> P. No, like to a gas station or something. Meet at a gas station. . . . dealers . . . just have a meeting place, "meet me here or meet me there." Or they will just come around and you know that somebody already called them before you did . . . and usually they have a pager or cell phone.

These examples illustrate the ways in which distributing and obtaining ecstasy occurs through social networks of friends who are selling and/or using it, and through social influence as dealers and users introduce others to the drug and try to convince them to use it and to share their experiences. They also illustrate the ways in which dealers and users develop relationships through which they seek safer and cheaper ways of obtaining a "quality high" and communicate about their experiences with other potential users. In this way they replicate the process that Kaufer and Carley refer to as constructuralism, where multiple and overlapping exchanges of similar messages occur among homophilous communicators with valued opinions (Kaufer & Carley, 1993).

Purchasing from Unknown Dealers in Clubs, Restaurants or Locations

Though most ecstasy is purchased from friends and personal dealers, some respondents reported purchasing ecstasy from sources they did not know well, a process that can be risky. One respondent, for example, said that he got ecstasy from different people. "I was willing to get it from the same person but you never know where the, because it is like, they get a pill and they gots different. It's like different things in them." He takes risks by buying ecstasy from people he doesn't know, but believes it is not possible to know what is in a pill by looking at it. Like other cautious users, his strategy for avoiding risk is to return to the same person if he has a good experience with a pill. Quality assurance is based on experience, which either reinforces and sustains a relationship between the customer and the dealer, or terminates it.

Some dealers prefer to sell in a club. They believe that it is safer because they are not exposed to the harassment and possible police arrest that they might encounter when selling on the street. There are, however, risks associated with selling inside a club, first from the house dealers (bouncers and bartenders or others approved for selling in the establishment), and second from police or investigators disguised as clients. For this reason, some prefer to act as brokers between the client and the dealer, carrying money from and drugs to the client. This role leaves them less exposed to arrest because they are not carrying more than one or two pills and their behavior is not as conspicuous. They can trade while appearing to be enjoying themselves at the club. They market ecstasy or other drugs by describing benefits to prospective clients, and can make money by "taxing" the product (i.e., adding a surcharge). Brokers are usually peers, similar to club attendees in age, ethnicity, style and appearance. They are motivated to promote the drugs since their profit depends on how much they sell.

One participant described how she obtained money from clients, got the pill, brought it to them and made a profit from the exchange.

> P. Whatever I felt like cutting (% tax), like an E pill, I would charge them thirty dollars for an E pill. Ten would be for me and twenty would go to the hustler . . . doing this, I was only in the club (meaning, she was acting like other club clients).
> I. So how would you find out how people would want some?
> P. 'Cause people are stupid and they would ask for it. . . . they would walk up and say "Yo you got E? Do you know who got the E, an you find me some." "Well, I can find you some E but it is going to cost you some." She argues, "We are in the club. It is late night. I don't know if you are undercover, I'm taking a risk. . . . they would be willing to accept my stories and willing to pay."

Thus she was able to tax whatever amount the market would bear. She was not afraid that they would not pay because as she put it, "we're in the same club, the club is not that big, you see my face, look at my face. If I don't come back, search for me, you're going to find me, I ain't leaving." In this case, the risk involved in obtaining the ecstasy became part of the marketing strategy.

Some dealers make their connections in the clubs, develop friendships and follow their clients to private parties.

> I. OK, now tell us about selling to you, which, which drug do you sell? Do you sell, some called street drugs, or have you sold like club drugs?
> P. I usually sell street drugs in the clubs. In the clubs, too, I just sell them on the streets but I switched from the street selling to clubs and parties . . . because (it's) less risky for one. You have the people there, the people get to know you better and you develop a friendship with the people that you're dealing with. So it's like a business, you know, a business-relationship slash friend-relationship so it's like . . . I meet you later at the party, so and so, I meet you there, you know what I'm saying.

Unlike the street situation, club-based sellers may try to exploit users who have no other means of procuring ecstasy, by overcharging the surcharge or "tax." For example, in one situation a club dealer tried to sell an ecstasy pill for $50.00 to users who did not know him. The clients were able to negotiate a better price, five pills for $90.00, but still considered this too much. Turning to another dealer, a friend of one of the group of youths, they were able to negotiate a better deal. When they described to the second dealer the attempt of the first dealer to sell pills at an exorbitant rate, he told them that the first dealer had obtained the pills from him, and that he had told the first dealer to elevate the cost by increasing the "tax." By giving a better price and appearing to be more honest and direct, the second dealer used the situation to compete with the first, and thus to obtain the loyalty and confidence of the buyers.

Obtaining Ecstasy at Private Parties

Ecstasy availability and use have been reported at private parties mainly held in hotel settings. Our researchers have obtained reports of private late-night or all-day hotel parties for the past several years. Entrance to these parties is through personal networks and ecstasy is widely used and usually available at approximately $20.00 a pill. Sometimes, marijuana is offered free until it is gone. When party attenders want more marijuana or are ready for ecstasy, it is available for a price. The association of ecstasy use with sexuality is the norm at these parties, and ecstasy use tends to be associated with group sex or sex with multiple partners.

In 2000, we received one report of a private "homework" party for middle school students from Hartford, at a home just outside of the city's southern boundary (in a safe "suburban" area) where the host's older siblings and their friends offered ecstasy to the students. There are no other examples of such parties but this technique is one that illustrates the important links between peri-urban and urban drug selling and use, and the way in which ecstasy dealers segment the market and the venue, and target their marketing strategies.

QUANTITATIVE EVIDENCE OF DIFFUSION OF ECSTASY INTO THE GENERAL POPULATION OVER TIME

To this point we have illustrated the primary mechanisms through which ecstasy is marketed and distributed, primarily through trusted and reliable personal networks, face-to-face (on the street) and electronically (via cell phone), and through personal networks or risk-taking homophilous and trusted dealers in club and party settings where ecstasy is marketed as "part of the scene."

Survey data from two studies illustrate the diffusion of ecstasy first among poly-drug users, and then into the general population. We began our surveys with poly-drug users between the ages of 16 and 24 in 1999 and continued through the end of 2000. In addition to age, eligibility for enrollment into our study was self-reported use of alcohol or any form of marijuana and any other drug in the previous 30 days. Recruiters were told specifically not to recruit for any specific additional drug. The recruitment procedure involved identifying qualified seeds, interviewing them and asking them to bring in members of their personal networks who met the enrollment criteria. For every participant referred by a seed who qualified, the seed received $5.00. Once our interest in ecstasy emerged, we took special care to monitor the recruitment process so as not to over-recruit ecstasy users. During the 17-month period from the start to finish of our baseline data collection period (May 1999-September, 2000), we saw a dramatic and statistically significant increase in reported use of ecstasy in our urban sample, as compared to other drugs.

To obtain these results, we segmented our baseline survey interviews by three-month periods (see Figure 1) from July 1999 to September 2000. This period corresponded to the process we have described earlier, in which ecstasy was diffusing from local clubs through club and friendship-based networks, into Hartford's neighborhoods.

When we compared rates across this time period for ecstasy against other drugs commonly used, only ecstasy showed a statistically significant increase in use across the designated time periods (.001). There were no significant differences in rate of reported use for any other of seven drugs (alcohol, marijuana, high THC marijuana, dust or PCP related substances, marijuana with additives, hallucinogens or cocaine).

Baseline data from our current study of transitions in club drug use, predictors and consequences,[3] (N = 555) collected during 2002-2003, shows a rate of approximately 25% use ever. The criteria for enrollment in this study are age (16-30) and, for RDS sampling, seeds must be residents of the city of Hartford. The sample is not recruited for any form of drug use and thus represents the general population of youths in that age group. The sample includes African American, Caribbean, Puerto Rican, other Latino and Caucasian male and female youth from locations throughout the city and surrounding towns. The ecstasy use rate is stable across a 12-month time period. The fact that the sample was recruited only by age and not by drug use and that the rate of ever-used has

FIGURE 1. Increases in Ecstasy Use Between June 1999 and September 2000

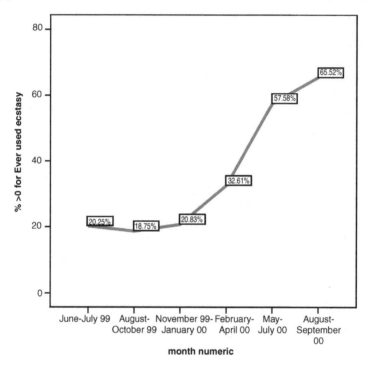

not changed over the period of the baseline study, suggests that ecstasy use has become normalized in the general population of urban youth at about 25% lifetime use. This is significantly higher than the highest annual prevalence, 11.4% of 12th grade users reported in Monitoring the Future (2002) at the peak of the ecstasy use curve, but it is important to remember that our sample consists of youth between 16 and 24, most of whom are likely to be at the peak of their drug-using careers.

DISCUSSION

Initially we argued that ecstasy, a new drug with pleasurable effects and few perceived short-term negative consequences, was diffused from suburban and "house" (bar and club-employed) dealers to urban youth who attended these locations. We proposed that homophily and trust were critical factors in the diffusion of ecstasy into urban networks and that direct and indirect social influence including specific market-ing strategies played an important role in encouraging people to initiate ecstasy use, and to continue it. It appears that the first significant en-counters of urban African American and Latino/Puerto Rican youth with ecstasy occurred in urban club settings. Thus it seems likely that young, primarily Puerto Rican, drug distributors first encountered, pur-chased and used ecstasy in Hartford's regular and after-hour clubs dur-ing events that mixed urban, suburban and college youth, and then began to market it to their friends as a new drug with positive results. It would be difficult to determine whether the introduction of ecstasy to urban African American and Latino/Puerto Rican youth occurred only as a result of their encounters with distributors in urban clubs. It may well be that large-scale urban distributors of cocaine or heroin were considering ways of priming the drug market for a new drug prior to the interaction of Puerto Rican and African American youth with suburban users and distributors in urban party settings, but we could not find evidence of this notion in our ethnographic data.

Ecstasy entered urban youth networks first through Latino youths who found it easier and perhaps more desirable than African Americans to mix in predominantly white party settings. Some of these youths were already involved in selling marijuana in these settings. They found it easy to share and promote the use of a new social drug with the capac-ity to support improved communication across personal and ethnic boundaries, to reduce tiredness after a long night out, and to enhance sensuality. For distributors, once the economic benefit and relative safety of selling ecstasy, in the form of easily hidden or destroyed pills, over marijuana became clear, it is likely that more youth turned to sell-ing and using ecstasy regularly in a variety of different settings. Users advertised the versatility of the new drug to their friends, and helped them to purchase it.

The role of the media to promote and diffuse information, beliefs and values regarding violence, drugs and, specifically, ecstasy, has been de-scribed elsewhere (Diamond, Bermudez, & Schensul, in review; Fan & Holway, 1994). Media promotion through music, videos, television shows, movies and performance, is effective as a form of "campaign" or "universal intervention." Ecstasy began to be promoted by African American Hip Hop/Rap artists in 2000-2001, most notably when Missy Elliot's album, "Miss (E) So Addictive" was first promoted at Urban Fashion Week in South Beach, Florida. The album's cover showing her with an ecstasy pill between her lips, clearly linked the music to the drug. Whether or not this moment, or the music referring to ecstasy use, has had a promotional effect on African American youth remains to be seen, since the music conveys mixed messages, and some of the artists who continue to sing about ecstasy are favored more among white than African American youth.

Regardless, creating a local market for a new drug involves identifying and targeting hidden, unique or special populations, and promoting use through social influence via trusted and effective role models who can frame positive messages about the drug, model use, assure safety and provide access at reasonable prices. In hidden populations, trusted agents or distributors who share like characteristics with users and engage with them regularly are in a strong position to influence them to try new drugs. The use of social marketing techniques in particular, price negotiation, and quality control and feedback, improves their capacity to expand their distribution system. Once they do so, continuous exchanges of information about the drug result in changing drug use norms, increased use, and an expanding drug market. This process is likely to be enhanced if it is supported by settings such as clubs or private parties that provide opportunity structures for use either by increasing access to drug purchasing, allowing use at the venue or promoting use through media messages or activities such as all-night dancing that benefit from its continued use.

CONCLUSIONS

Agar's model accounting for the introduction and evolution of new drug trends refers to the market, the distributors and a large-scale event or change in an established system of drug distribution (Agar & Reisinger, 2003). In his macrolevel model, a rearrangement of global distributors interfaced with a waiting market, youths involved in raves and all-night dance events and the settings created for them by entrepreneurial promoters. This model is useful for explaining the infrastructure that supports the global and national availability of new drugs. But it does not explain the mechanisms through which norms, practices, and products diffuse through local markets. Diffusion models provide effective ways of understanding and interpreting local behaviors identified through a combination of qualitative and quantitative data on new drug practices. The first markets for ecstasy (like heroin, cocaine and marijuana) were those with monied-middle-class suburban youth able to spend substantial amounts of money on a drug that made them feel good on the weekend with few perceived short-term side effects. Once this market was saturated, distributors turned to uninformed urban youth, targeting first those Latino youth able to mingle in white environments and desiring to emulate the material goods and cultural life-style of middle class white professionals, and then the broader urban market. As with other products marketed to groups experiencing economic disparities, drug prices adjust to the market. In the case of ecstasy, these adjustments are made primarily through adulterating and diluting products. Unfortunately, because MDMA is a scheduled drug, and because young inner city youth and young adults do not, for the most part, use the internet to monitor drug trends and dangers, they have no way of knowing what they are ingesting except by trying it or watching others use it. Fortunately, most ecstasy adulterants and fillers tend to be caffeine, sugar and starch-based; thus, clients may be disappointed but generally they do not die or become addicted. More research is needed to determine ways that urban youths participate in and are influenced by large-scale marketing schemes that promote the use of new products including drugs, and how, with limited resources, they cope with the changing quality of new products.

NOTES

1. NIDA Grant # R01 DA11421, PI: J. Schensul, entitled *Pathways to High Risk Drug Use Among Urban Youth.*
2. In all instances, "P" refers to participant, "I" refers to interviewer.
3. NIDA Grant # DA 01 010, PI. J. Schensul, *Club Drugs, Resource Inequities and Social Health.*

REFERENCES

Agar, M., & Reisinger, H. S. (2003). Going for the global: The case of ecstasy. *Human Organization, 62* (1), 1-11.
Bearison, D. J. (1982). New directions in studies of social interaction and cognitive growth. In F. C. Serafica (Ed.), *Social-cognitive development in context* (pp. 199-221). New York: Guilford Press.
Bellis, M. A., Hughes, K., Bennett, A., & Thomson, R. (2003). The role of an international nightlife resort in the proliferation of recreational drugs, *Addiction* (Vol. 98, pp. 1713-1721).
Berger, P. L., & Luckmann, T. (1966). *The social construction of reality: A treatise in the sociology of knowledge* (1st ed.). Garden City, NY: Doubleday.
Black, D., Blue, C. L., & Coster, D. C. (2001). Using social marketing to develop and test tailored health messages. *American Journal of Health Behavior* (Vol. 25, pp. 260-271).

Boyd, C. J., McCabe, S. E., & d'Arcy, H. (2003). Ecstasy use among college undergraduates: Gender, race and sexual identity. *Journal of Substance Abuse Treatment, 24* (3), 209-215.

Brecht, M. L., & von Mayrhauser, C. (2002). Differences between Ecstasy-using and non-using methamphetamine users. *Journal of Psychoactive Drugs* (Vol. 34, pp. 215-223).

Breslau, K. (2002). The 'sextasy' craze. Clubland's dangerous party mix: Viagra and ecstasy. *Newsweek, 139* (22), 30.

Calafat, A., Fernández, C., Juan, M., Bellis, M. A., Bohrn, K., Hakkarainen, P. et al. (2001). *Risk and control in the recreational drug culture.* Palma de Mallorca: Irefrea.

Calafat, A., & Stocco, P. (2000). Recreational life and ecstasy use. In J. Fountain (Ed.), *Understanding and responding to drug use: The role of qualitative research. EMCDDA Scientific Monograph Series (N°4).* Luxembourg: Office for Official Publications of the European Communities.

Colfax, G. N., Mansergh, G., Guzman, R., Vittinghoff, E., Marks, G., Rader, M. et al. (Writer) (2001). Drug use and sexual risk behavior among gay and bisexual men who attend circuit parties: A venue-based comparison, *Journal of Acquired Immune Deficiency Syndromes.*

Diamond, S., Bermudez, R., & Schensul, J. (In review). What's the rap about ecstasy?: Popular song lyrics and drug trends among American youth. *Journal of Adolescent Research.*

Donaldson, S. I., Graham, J. W., & Hansen, W. B. (1994). Testing the generalizability of intervening mechanism theories: Understanding the effects of adolescent drug-use prevention interventions. *Journal of Behavioral Medicine, 17* (2), 195-216.

Eiserman, J., Singer, M., Schensul, J., & Broomhall, L. (2003). Methodological challenges in club drug research. *Practicing Anthropology, 25* (3), 19-22.

Elliott, L., Morrison, A., Ditton, J., Farrall, S., Short, E., Cowan, L. et al. (1998). *Alcohol, drug use and sexual behavior of young adults on a Mediterranean dance holiday.*

Fan, D. P., & Holway, W. B. (1994). Media coverage of cocaine and its impact on usage patterns. *International Journal of Public Opinion Research, 6* (2), 139-162.

Fitzgerald, J., & Hamilton, M. (1994). *An exploratory study of hallucinogen use in Melbourne.* University of Melbourne, Melbourne.

Flocks, J., Clarke, L., Albrecht, S., Bryant, C., Monaghan, P., & Baker, H. (2001). Implementing a community-based social marketing project to improve agricultural worker health. *Environmental Health Perspectives, 109* (Suppl 3), 461-468.

Forsyth, A. J. M. (1996). Places and patterns of drug use in the Scottish dance scene. *Addiction, 91* (4), 511-521.

Forsyth, A. J. M., Barnard, M., & McKeganey, N. P. (1997). Musical preference as an indicator of adolescent drug use. *Addiction, 92* (10), 1317-1325.

Friedman, S. R., DesJarlais, D. C., & Ward, T. P. (1994). Social models for changing health-relevant behavior. In R. J. DiClemente & J. L. Peterson (Eds.), *Preventing AIDS: Theories and methods of behavioral interventions* (pp. 95-116). New York: Plenum Press.

Guisinger, S., & Blatt, S. J. (1994). Individuality and relatedness: Evolution of a fundamental dialectic. *American Psychologist, 49* (2), 104-111.

Harter, S. (1990a). Developmental differences in the nature of self-representations: Implications for the understanding, assessment, and treatment of maladaptive behavior. *Cognitive Therapy & Research, 14* (2), 113-142.

Harter, S. (1990b). Self and identity development. In S. S. Feldman & G. R. Elliott (Eds.), *At the threshold: The developing adolescent* (pp. 352-387). Cambridge, MA: Harvard University Press.

Hawkins, J., Hill, K. G., Guo, J., & Battin-Pearson, S. R. (2002). Substance use norms and transitions in substance use: Implications for the Gateway Hypothesis. In D. B. Kandel (Ed.), *Stages and pathways of drug involvement: Examining the Gateway Hypothesis* (pp. 42-64). New York, NY: Cambridge University Press.

Hunt, G., & Evans, K. (2003). Dancing and drugs: A cross-national perspective. *Contemporary Drug Problems, 30* (4), 779-814.

Kaufer, D. S., & Carley, K. M. (1993). *Communication at a distance: The effect of print on socio-cultural organization and change.* Hillsdale, NJ: Lawrence Erlbaum Associates.

Latané, B., Liu, J. H., Nowak, A., Bonevento, M., & Zheng, L. (1995). Distance matters–physical space and social impact. *Personality and Social Psychology Bulletin, 21* (8), 795-805.

Latané, B., Nowak, A., & Liu, J. H. (1994). Measuring emergent social phenomena-dynamism, polarization, and clustering as order parameters of social-systems. *Behavioral Science, 39* (1), 1-24.

Latané, B. B. (1995). Minority influence and dynamic social impact. *Review of Social Psychology* (Vol. 10, pp. 105-109).

Latkin, C. A. (1995). A personal network approach to AIDS prevention: An experimental peer group intervention for street-injecting drug users: The SAFE study. *NIDA Research Monograph, 151*, 181-195.

Lee, S. J., Galanter, M., Dermatis, H., & McDowell, D. (Eds.) (2003). Circuit parties and patterns of drug use in a subset of gay men. *Journal of Addictive Diseases* 22(4): 47-60.

Lenton, S., Boys, A., & Norcross, K. (1997). Raves, drugs and experience: Drug use by a sample of people who attend raves in Western Australia. *Addiction, 92* (10), 1327-1337.

Lewis, L. A., & Ross, M. W. (1995). The gay dance party culture in Sydney: A qualitative analysis. *Journal of Homosexuality, 29* (1), 113-142.

Mattison, A. M., Ross, M. W., Wolfson, T., Franklin, D., & San Diego, H. I. V. N. R. C. G. (2001). Circuit party attendance, club drug use, and unsafe sex in gay men. *Journal of Substance Abuse* (Vol. 13, pp. 119-126).

Maxwell, J. C. (2003). The response to club drug use. *Current Opinion in Psychiatry, 16* (3), 279-289.

Maxwell, J. C. (2004). *Patterns of club drug use in the U.S., 2004: Ecstasy, GHB, Ketamine, LSD, Methamphetamine, Rohypnol.* Austin, TX: The Center for Excellence in Drug Epidemiology, The Gulf Coast Addiction Technology Transfer Center, The University of Texas at Austin.

Maxwell, K. A. (2002). Friends: The role of peer influence across adolescent risk behaviors. *Journal of Youth & Adolescence, 31* (4), 267-277.

Merchant, J., & Macdonald, R. (1994). Youth and rave culture, ecstasy and health. *Youth and Policy: The Journal of Critical Analysis, 45*, 16-38.

Newmeyer, J. A., Feldman, H. W., Biernacki, P., & Watters, J. K. (1989). Preventing AIDS contagion among intravenous drug users. *Medical Anthropology, 10* (2-3), 167-175.

Nowak, A., Szamrej, J., & Latane, B. (1990). From private attitude to public-opinion– A dynamic theory of social impact. *Psychological Review, 97* (3), 362-376.

Parker, H., Aldridge, J., & Measham, F. (1998). Illegal leisure: The normalization of adolescent recreational drug use. London & New York: Routledge.

Riley, S. C. E., & Hayward, E. (2004). Patterns, trends, and meanings of drug use by dance-drug users in Edinburgh, Scotland. *Drugs-Education Prevention and Policy, 11* (3), 243-262.

Rogoff, B. (2003). *The cultural nature of human development.* New York: Oxford University Press.

Romanelli, F., Smith, K. M., & Pomeroy, C. (2003). Use of club drugs by HIV-seropositive and HIV-seronegative gay and bisexual men. *Topics in HIV Medicine* (Vol. 11, pp. 25-32).

Ross, M. W., Mattison, A. M., & Franklin, D. R. (Cartographer) (2003). Club drugs and sex on drugs are associated with different motivations for gay circuit party attendance in men. *Substance Use and Misuse 38*(8): 1173-1183

Sale, E. W. (1999). *Toward an integrative model of substance use among high-risk youth populations.* University of Missouri-Saint Louis, US, 1.

Schensul, J. J. (2001, July 20). *The diffusion of MDMA use among urban youth in Hartford, CT: Implications for drug and HIV prevention in club drug users and their networks.* Paper presented at the NIDA Conference, Ecstasy: MDMA/Ecstasy research: Advances, challenges, future directions, Bethesda, MD.

Schensul, J. J., Huebner, C., Singer, M., Snow, M., Feliciano, P., & Broomhall, L. (2000). The high, the money, and the fame: The emergent social context of "new marijuana" use among urban youth. *Medical Anthropology, 18* (4), 389-414.

Singer, M., & Weeks, M. R. (1992). *Hartford Target Sampling Plan: Community Alliance for AIDS Programs.* Hartford, CT: Hispanic Health Council.

Solowij, N., Hall, W., & Lee, N. (1992). Recreational MDMA use in Sydney: A profile of 'Ecstacy' users and their experiences with the drug. *British Journal of Addiction, 87* (8), 1161-1172.

Tong, T., & Boyer, E. W. (2002). Club drugs, smart drugs, raves, and circuit parties: An overview of the club scene. *Pediatric Emergency Care* (Vol. 18, pp. 216-218).

Vygotsky, L. S. (1978). *Mind in society: The development of higher psychological processes.* Cambridge: Harvard University Press.

Wallace, J. M., Jr., Bachman, J. G., O'Malley, P. M., Johnston, L. D., Schulenberg, J. E., & Cooper, S. M. (2002). Tobacco, alcohol, and illicit drug use: Racial and ethnic differences among U.S. high school seniors, 1976-2000. *Public Health Reports, 117* (Supplement 1), S67-75.

Watters, J. K., & Biernacki, P. (1989). Targeted sampling: Options for the study of hidden populations. *Social Problems, 36* (4), 416-430.

Weir, E. (2000). Raves: A review of the culture, the drugs and the prevention of harm [see comment] *CMAJ Canadian Medical Association Journal* (Vol. 162, pp. 1843-1848).

Wertsch, J. V. (1991). *Voices of the mind: A sociocultural approach to mediated action.* Cambridge, MA: Harvard University Press.

Yacoubian, G. S. (2003). Tracking ecstasy trends in the United States with data from three national drug surveillance systems. *Journal of Drug Education* (Vol. 33, pp. 245-258).

Yacoubian, G. S., Jr. (2002a). Assessing the temporal relationship between race and ecstasy use among high school seniors. *Journal of Drug Education* (Vol. 32, pp. 213-225).

Yacoubian, G. S., Jr. (2002b). Correlates of Ecstasy use among tenth graders surveyed through monitoring the future. *Journal of Psychoactive Drugs* (Vol. 34, pp. 225-230).

Yacoubian, G. S., Jr. (2003). Correlates of ecstasy use among students surveyed through the 1997 College Alcohol Study. *Journal of Drug Education* (Vol. 33, pp. 61-69).

Yacoubian, G. S., Jr., Arria, A. M., Fost, E., & Wish, E. D. (2002). Estimating the prevalence of Ecstasy use among juvenile offenders. *Journal of Psychoactive Drugs* (Vol. 34, pp. 209-213).

Yacoubian, G. S., Jr., Boyle, C., Harding, C. A., & Loftus, E. A. (2003). It's a rave new world: Estimating the prevalence and perceived harm of ecstasy and other drug use among club rave attendees. *Journal of Drug Education* (Vol. 33, pp. 187-196).

When the Drug of Choice
Is a Drug of Confusion:
Embalming Fluid Use
in Inner City Hartford, CT

Merrill Singer, PhD
Greg Mirhej, MA
Susan Shaw, PhD
Hassan Saleheen, MD
James Vivian, PhD

Dr. Merrill Singer is Director of Research at the Center for Community Health Research of the Hispanic Health Council and Principal Investigator on the CDC-funded Building Community Responses to Risks of Emergent Drug Use project.

Greg Mirhej is Project Coordinator of the Building Community Responses project.

Dr. Susan Shaw, who served as initial Project Coordinator on the Building Community Responses project, is Senior Researcher at the Hispanic Health Council.

Dr. Hassan Saleheen is Data Analyst on the Building Community Responses project.

Dr. James Vivian is Chief Data Analyst at the Hispanic Health Council.

Erica Hastings is Evaluator of the intervention component of the Building Community Responses project.

Lucy Rohena is Outreach/Interviewer on the Building Community Responses project.

DeShawn Jennings is Outreach/Interviewer on the Building Community Responses project.

Juhem Navarro is Data Manager on the Building Community Responses project.

Claudia Santelices is Ethnographer on the Building Community Responses project.

Dr. Alan H. B. Wu is Professor of Laboratory Medicine, University of California, San Francisco.

Andrew Smith is Laboratory Technician at the University of California, San Francisco.

Dr. Alberto Perez is Assistant Clinical Professor in the Department of Emergency Medicine, University of Connecticut School of Medicine and the Division of Medical Toxicology, Department of Traumatology and Emergency Medicine, Hartford Hospital.

Address correspondence to: Merrill Singer, PhD, Hispanic Health Council, 175 Main Street, Hartford, CT 06106 (E-mail: anthro8566@aol.com).

[Haworth co-indexing entry note]: "When the Drug of Choice Is a Drug of Confusion: Embalming Fluid Use in Inner City Hartford, CT." Singer, Merrill et al. Co-published simultaneously in *Journal of Ethnicity in Substance Abuse* (The Haworth Press, Inc.) Vol. 4, No. 2, 2005, pp. 73-96; and: *New Drugs on the Street: Changing Inner City Patterns of Illicit Consumption* (ed: Merrill Singer) The Haworth Press, Inc., 2005, pp. 73-96. Single or multiple copies of this article are available for a fee from The Haworth Document Delivery Service [1-800-HAWORTH, 9:00 a.m. - 5:00 p.m. (EST). E-mail address: docdelivery@haworthpress.com].

doi:10.1300/J233v04n02_04

73

Erica Hastings, MA
Lucy Rohena
DeShawn Jennings
Juhem Navarro, MA
Claudia Santelices, MA, PhD (cand.)
Alan H. B. Wu, PhD
Andrew Smith, MA
Alberto Perez, MD

SUMMARY. This paper examines the use of a new illicit drug–embalming fluid mixtures–in Hartford, CT based on a recent assessment of drug consumption in an outreach-recruited sample of 242 not-in-treatment active drug users. Sociodemographic, drug use, and health and social problems of drug users who do and do not use embalming fluid mixture are presented, revealing some notable differences between these two groups of street drug users. Despite regular consumption, we report that embalming fluid mixture users are often uncertain about what is in this new drug, despite experiencing often powerful effects. Urine toxicology findings from a subsample of individuals who used embalming fluid mixtures in the last 48 hours, reveal the frequent presence of phencyclidine (PCP) as well as other drugs. The public health implications of this new wave of PCP use are assessed. *[Article copies available for a fee from The Haworth Document Delivery Service: 1-800-HAWORTH. E-mail address: <docdelivery@haworthpress.com> Website: <http://www.HaworthPress. com> © 2005 by The Haworth Press, Inc. All rights reserved.]*

KEYWORDS. Embalming fluid, phencyclidine, substance abuse, public health

In the last several years, there have been various reports of the use of embalming fluid as a psychoactive drug, especially among urban youth (Elwood, 1998; Holland et al., 1998). Despite indications that in some locations, including our own research site in Hartford, CT (Singer et al., 2000; Singer et al., in press (a)), this drug has become very popular among younger street drug users (and to a lesser degree older drug users as well), there remains considerable uncertainty as to its exact chemical composition. This fact is reflected in the diversity of street names used for the substance, e.g., "dust," "wet," "tecal," "illy," "matrix," and "fry" among others, not just nationally but within the same city. Reports of embalming fluid mixture use as a mood/mind-altering drug date as far back as the 1980s (Spector, 1985; James and Johnson, 1996), although the extent of ethnographic research on this drug continues to be quite limited. Some researchers (e.g., Holland et al., 1998) and a number of websites linked to the term "embalming fluid" argue that this drug is nothing other than PCP (phencyclidine) wrapped in a new guise by drug producers in order to attract a new market for an old drug. For example, the Vaults of Erowid website, an online library of information about psychoactive plants and chemicals frequented primarily by younger drug users (http://www.erowid.org/chemicals/pcp/pcp_info6.shtml), reports the following:

> [This drug is] sold in a variety of forms including cannabis joints or regular cigarettes dipped in liquid and cannabis leaf or tea leaves dipped in liquid. In all of these forms, the material is then smoked. Despite the variety of names, there is good reason to believe that these are all various preparations containing PCP. In most instances PCP is not mentioned when the substance is sold or discussed. In fact, there are constantly recirculating rumors that substances being sold by these names do not contain PCP, but are instead actually the fluid (formaldehyde) used for embalming as would be used in a mortuary. But there is evidence to support that this is primarily a case of confused slang terms. "Embalming Fluid" is a common street slang term for PCP and has been for many years. PCP can come in liquid form, so the term "fluid" is fitting. It is entirely possible (actually quite likely) that the confusion between PCP and embalming fluid (formaldehyde) has gone so far as to cause a new trend where PCP is actually mixed with formaldehyde (or other "embalming fluids") and used as a recreational psychoactive. But there is little evidence that the formaldehyde itself causes any pleasant or desirable effects.

As this statement makes clear, a new drug (or an old drug with a new label) is now growing in popularity, but despite the certainty expressed at the erowid website, its actual contents continue to be argued by researchers, users, and even those who sell and use the drug. If PCP is gaining a new generation of adherents who do not know they are using the drug, this is of considerable public health concern.

Developed in the 1950s and initially used medically as a general anesthetic, the medical use of PCP was rapidly discontinued when it was observed that between 10-30% of recipients exhibited post-operative psychoses and dysphoria (Peters and Stillman, 1978). The drug continues to be used in veterinary medicine, and theft from veterinary clinics is one source of supply for illicit use. PCP first appeared as a street drug in San Francisco in 1967. Even at that time it was sold under the names of various popular hallucinogens, such as LSD, MDA, mescaline, and THC. Nonetheless, PCP quickly gained a reputation for often causing bad reactions among users (Farber et al., 2003; Hoaken and Stewart, 2003). While a single exposure to PCP frightens many people into never knowingly using it again, others report enjoying the PCP experience, including its reported ability to produce feelings of strength, power, invulnerability, and a mental numbing sensation. Many PCP users wind up in emergency rooms because of overdose or because of the drug's upsetting psychological effects. In a hospital or detention setting, these people often become violent. The drug has been linked to violence in other settings as well, such as homeless shelters and on the street (Lerner and Burns, 1978; Mokhlesi et al., 2004; Wish, 1986). The sedative properties of PCP, in interaction with other central nervous system depressants such as alcohol and benzodiazepines, can lead to blackouts and coma. Nonetheless, 14% of young adults reported PCP use in 1978 (U.S. Department of Health and Human Services, 1979). Metabolism in the body is known to slow with habitual use, and regular PCP users can experience symptoms of the high days after use. Ironically, given its frequent association with violence, the drug was once sold on the street as the "PeaCe Pill."

During this early period of use, PCP consumption was documented by the Drug Enforcement Administration in a number of major U.S. cities, including Chicago, Miami, New York City, and Philadelphia. Despite its initial rise in popularity, as is common in the "life history" of psychotropic drugs, PCP use subsequently waned throughout the 1970s (Singer, in press); although sporadic reports of renewed use have appeared over time.

Over time, PCP has retained a covert quality, appearing under diverse names, inserted in ready-made drug mixtures, and often sold as other substances. From a public health standpoint, uncertainty about a drug's chemical makeup is particularly problematic because appropriate response requires a clear understanding of the health problems being addressed. In this light, the purpose of this paper is to report new findings on the use of "embalming fluid mixtures" in Hartford and the dilemmas this drug has created in attempting to build an evidenced-based community response to emergent drug use trends. Specifically, this paper assesses experience, knowledge and attitudes about embalming fluid use in a sample of 242 active street drug users, including a comparison of the sociodemographic and other characteristics of recent users (within the last 30 days) and non-users of embalming fluid mixture. Highlighted in this assessment is the considerable level of uncertainty about the contents of the drug. To address this issue, we also report findings from a laboratory test of the urine of individuals who reported recent (last 48 hours) use of the drug and analysis. Based on this information the paper addresses the public health challenges in an emerging drug use epidemic when there is considerable uncertainty among users and researchers alike about drug contents.

METHODS

The data reported in this paper were collected through the Centers for Disease Control and Prevention (CDC)-funded Building Community Responses to Risks of Emergent Drug Use project in Hartford, CT. This project was designed to collect three waves of survey data on emergent and changing patterns of street drug use, as well as accompanying ethnographic observational and unstructured interview data associated with each wave of the survey. The data reported here are from the second wave of data collection which was carried out from April 15 to August 26, 2004. Survey data are reported for 242 individuals. Criteria for participating in the survey included a minimum age of 18, use of illicit drugs during the last 30 days, and no participation in any self-help/ 12-step groups or admission to drug treatment or detoxification in the last 30 days.

The survey instrument used in this project was a modified version of the *AIDS Risk Assessment (ARA)*. This instrument, originally developed by Mark Williams for use with drug users in Houston, is a shortened version of the Risk Behavior Assessment developed and widely used and validated by NIDA. Data were collected on a range of variables that included sociodemographic characteristics, historic and current drug use patterns, attitudes and knowledge about specific drugs of interest, drug-related health and social consequences experienced by participants, and awareness of emergent and changing drug use practice locally. The survey was administered by trained project staff in interview rooms at the Hispanic Health Council.

Participants for this study were recruited through street outreach (Singer et al., 2000). Procedures used for the recruitment and interviewing of participants are as follows:

1. Outreach workers, who were matched to the target population of street drug users by gender, language, and ethnicity, were trained in: target group and target area identification, street approach and engagement strategies, rapport-building, conflict de-escalation, human subject issues, street safety, and participant screening and intake procedures.

2. Outreach workers began work in a target neighborhood–identified in prior research as high drug use areas–by visiting known community agencies, service providers, shelters, churches, neighborhood stores, and community police, assigned to the target neighborhoods, to introduce themselves and begin to become familiar (or for seasoned outreach workers, more familiar) in the target neighborhoods.

3. The project also was advertised through local African American, Latino, Gay/Lesbian community newspapers, as well as through public service announcement on local radio stations, on college bulletin boards, and at community health clinics.

4. Outreach workers introduced the project and explained its objectives to potential participants and assessed them in terms of meeting project inclusion criteria and willingness to participate. Candidate participants who passed this screening process were given an appointment card to participate in the project survey interview, as well as specific directions and a map to the Hispanic Health Council, and a bus token. Participants were told that if they were unable to make their interview appointment, to contact the outreach worker by phone to set up another appointment.

5. Upon arrival at their appointed interview, candidate participants were re-screened in terms of project inclusion criteria, consented for participation in the project survey, and interviewed by a project interviewer.

6. At the end of their survey interview, some participants–based on a plan designed to recruit a gender, ethnic and age mixture that reflected the larger sample, as well as exhibiting a willingness to be open and talkative–were invited to participate in the in-depth interview component of the study. The 35 individuals who were recruited for this component were given a follow-up interview appointment with either the project ethnographer or project coordinator, both of whom conducted these qualitative interviews (with open-ended questions). These interviews were intended to provide detailed, personal accounts of life and drug use history, contemporary consumption patterns, drug understand-

ings and attitudes, contexts of drug use, experiences of drug use, and health and social consequences of involvement with illicit drugs. Following subject consent, qualitative interviews–which were guided by a set of interview questions but allowed to flow as participants talked about specific issues of concern or interest to them or were asked clarifying probe questions–were tape recorded, translated (if conducted in Spanish), transcribed, and coded for key themes relative to the project goals of tracing emergent and changing drug use practice in the city. The project ethnographer also conducted street observation in drug use areas and accompanied drug users to use sites to observe drug use, including embalming fluid use, with a handful of participants. Qualitative interviews were also conducted with health care and drug treatment providers and other individuals who worked professionally with drug using populations and might have knowledge of changing drug use practices, populations, or risks.

Additionally, 30 survey participants who reported the use of embalming fluid mixtures during the last 48 hours were recruited to participate in the laboratory assay component of the study. These individuals were escorted to the laboratory room at the Hispanic Health Council (which resembles a clinical examining room with adjacent bathroom connected by a window to transmit urine samples). Participants were asked a series of questions about recent drug use and related issues to flag known confounders in urine drug assay. Urine samples, in standard collection cups, were refrigerated and transported at regular intervals to the clinical chemistry laboratory at Hartford Hospital. The urine was tested for drugs of abuse using a commercial immunoassay called Triage (Biosite Diagnostics, San Diego, CA). Samples were tested for major metabolites of PCP, cocaine, marijuana, and heroin.

Participants were paid a $20 incentive for completing a survey interview and $20 for completing a qualitative interview or providing a urine sample. Drug users who requested drug treatment, medical services, social services or other types of intervention during outreach, participation in the survey, or participation in the qualitative interview or toxicological sample collection, were referred to the appropriate service provider.

EMBALMING FLUID MIXTURE USERS

Of the 242 active drug users recruited in the second wave of the project survey, 99 (41%) participants reported ever using embalming fluid mixtures, while 42 (17%) reported the use of this drug during the last 30 days. Reasons for not continuing the use of embalming fluid mixtures varied, but for many individuals their decision was shaped by particularly unpleasant or frightening experiences with the drug. As one female participant explained:

> I've done dust once and I told my boyfriend I'll never do it again. I've no [extensive] experience of dust. I just know that I had a friend who got high a couple of years ago and he was so messed up! He [did] not even know his own name . . . Seriously, he would not even be able to drive his car home . . . I'm scared of dust.

It is the group of recent embalming fluid mixture users (EFMU), those who have used the drug during the last 30 days, who are examined primarily in this paper. These individuals were recruited from 12 of the 15 Hartford neighborhoods where individuals from the total sample were recruited. Notably, 50% of the EFMU were recruited from just three contiguous neighborhoods on the south end of the city, an area that is predominantly Latino (with Puerto Ricans comprising the majority of Latinos in these neighborhoods). Indeed, Latinos comprised 52% of the individuals who reported embalming fluid use during the last 30 days (while accounting for 40% of the non-EFMU in our sample). While roughly equal percentages of African Americans are found in the EFMU and non-EFMU subgroups (31% and 33% respectively), white participants were significantly more likely not to be users of embalming fluid mixtures (non-EFMU = 22%, EFMU = 10%). Additionally, individuals who ever used embalming fluid mixture as well as those who used it in the last 30 days were more likely to be male than female ($p < .05$).

We did not find any significant differences in terms of employment status of EFMU and other drug users in the sample; the majority of all participants in the sample were unemployed (69% among EFMU and 72% non-EFMU respectively) and only a small percentage of participants reported full-time employment (7% and 8% respectively). A little over one-third of users and non-users of embalming fluid mixtures considered themselves to be homeless (36% and 37% respectively). While most participants were poor, whatever their drug use pattern, the EFMU tended to be somewhat poorer than those who did not use embalming fluid mixtures, with 76% of the former compared to 62% of the latter reporting less than $1000/month in total income. EFMU were also more likely to derive income through drug sales than those who did not use this drug (23% vs. 10% respectively) and somewhat more likely to report "hustling" as an income source (45% vs. 37% respectively), while welfare or disability was most often the source of income for those participants who did not use embalming fluid mixtures. To some degree, the characteristics reported above reflect the fact that the EFMU tended to be younger than other members of the sample (with a mean age of 28 years for EFMU compared to 34 years for the whole sample, p < .05), confirming our prior findings that embalming fluid users tend to be younger, on average, than the general population of street drug users (Singer et al., in press(a); Singer, in press). As one participant in the study noted:

> All the young kids [in the neighborhood are using embalming fluid]. Oh my god! More Puerto Rican and Black [kids]. . . . It's a teenage thing. The guys are 20 something, 25, 26 and down.

The comparative age ranges of participants who have used or not used embalming fluid mixtures in the last 30 days, as reported in Table 1, confirm this participant's statement.

Table 1 also reflects, however, a growing diffusion of embalming fluid mixture use beyond younger users to those over the age of 30, especially to those in the 30-40 age bracket. As we have argued elsewhere (Singer, in press), one common drug use dynamic is "diversification," the spread in the use of a particular drug among social networks that comprise different ethnic, age, lifestyle, cultural, regional, or identity groups with otherwise differing drug use patterns. Illicit drugs that diversify tend to have longer-term waves of use in a population. Those that remain concentrated in only one group of users tend to exhibit diminished use over time as the user group changes (e.g., as youth age or as an ethnic group improves its social status in society). Because drug distribution is driven by profit-seeking, diminished use of a drug at one point in time does not mean the drug will not "return," perhaps in a new guise or as part of a drug mixture.

TABLE 1. Age Ranges of Participants

	18-24 yrs	26-30 yrs	31-40 yrs	41+ yrs
Embalming fluid mixture users	45%	21%	29%	5%
Non-users of embalming fluid	32%	8%	31%	30%

The mean age at first use of embalming fluid mixtures among our participants was 20.6 years. Almost a third (29%) of EFMU said that they, in turn, have introduced others to the drug. EFMU reported that all (21%) or most (21%) of their friends use embalming fluid mixtures (compared to 7% and 4% respectively among non-EFMU). Friends of EFMU, however, were most likely to use marijuana, with 74% of our participants reporting that all of their friends use marijuana. Among non-users of embalming fluid mixtures, by contrast, only 43% reported that all of their friends use marijuana. Responding to a question about his initiation into embalming fluid use, for example, one of our participants stated:

> A: Like, I guess I was smoking marijuana so long it wasn't affecting me anymore, . . . it was just like cigarettes basically, so I just tried something new . . . [S]ome of my other friends were doing this thing called illy, it was called illy at the time because it wasn't called dust yet, so . . . I decided to smoke some just to try it. At first I didn't like it because the high was like, it made you feel like real paranoid, and then the second time I tried it I liked it, so ever since I've been smoking it off and on. . . . [T]he first time I didn't like it because it made me hallucinate.
> Q: So what kind of things did you see?
> A: Like, the grim reaper and I seen like different color cats just running past . . . it makes your pupils dilate real big and you just see a whole bunch of things and you can't really walk.

EFMU reported that, on average, they used embalming fluid on seven of the previous 30 days. During this period, they spent about $300 a week on drugs (i.e., on all the drugs they used, not just embalming fluid mixtures), which they indicated was a typical weekly drug expense for them. Most of the EFMU in our sample usually acquired embalming fluid mixture on the street from a drug dealer. Eighty-four percent said that embalming fluid mixtures were either "very easy" or "easy" to get on the street; only 2% reported that the drug was hard to get.

The drug is sold in a limited number of locations around the city according to participants and our field observations, often as a black powder that can be in a cigar which has been cut open, or a cigarette wrapping paper for smoking. It is also sold in a liquid form that is dripped on to a smokable leaf (e.g., marijuana or mint). The majority of EFMU also reported that after acquiring the drug they tend to use it at home or in someone else's home rather than on the street or in an abandoned building (which is common among drug injectors and crack cocaine users).

Some of our study participants were able to fully describe the preparation process for turning embalming fluid mixture into a consumable drug. One explained that when combined with mint leaves, the process of production involves heating the plant leaves in a microwave oven until they turn dark black, and then sprinkling the embalming fluid on them. The mint absorbs the fluid, we were told, turning it into a black dusty substance that is then poured into a blunt cigar that is split open, filled, and then re-wrapped. Dipping tobacco cigarettes directly into a jar of embalming fluid prior to smoking also occurs according to a number of the individuals we interviewed. Several participants reported that dry forms of the drug are manufactured by soaking leaves (marijuana, mint or tea leaves) in embalming fluid and freezing them. Freezing apparently acts as a dehydrator, and the leaves are crumbled to make a dry black powder, which is bagged, sold on the street, and sprinkled by the consumer into cigars or marijuana cigarettes. The substance is recognizable to drug users by its appearance and smell. As one participant explained:

Q: You've seen a bag of dust?
A: Yeah it's black, and with the nastiest smell . . .
Q: Everybody talks about the chemical smell.
A: Yeah, it is horrible . . . I don't know, it smells like something they put in dead people . . . You can smell it on you if you smoke it.

Another participant told us:

[Wet] comes in a little glass bottle. My friend used it to dip [blunt cigars]. It stinks when you smoke it.

We found that the EFMU in our sample tended to be poly-drug users. In fact, less than a fourth of the EFMU that we interviewed (23%) indicated that of the various drugs they use, embalming fluid mixtures gave them the greatest pleasure. While the favorite drugs of non-EFMU were heroin (40% of non-EFMU), crack/cocaine (28%), and marijuana (22%), among EFMU the favorite drugs were heroin (26%), marijuana (26%), and embalming fluid mixture (23%). Table 2 reports the other drugs used by EFMU during the last 30 days in comparison with the non-EFMU in our sample. With reference to two drugs, ecstasy and heroin, there were significant differences between EFMU and non-EFMU in prevalence of use. Age differences between these two groups may be a factor in these different drug use patterns, as ecstasy, like embalming fluid mixture, tends to be a youth drug. At any rate, Table 2 reveals that EFMU tend to be heavy drug users overall with illicit consumption of a broad range of other street drugs in addition to embalming fluid mixtures.

DRUG-RELATED HEALTH AND SOCIAL PROBLEMS AMONG EFMU

Although he is from Connecticut, Billie Smith was not a participant in our study, but he easily could have been. Like the majority of our study participants, he was an inner city, gang-involved youth who smoked marijuana. On September 4, 1994, and on the previous evening,

TABLE 2. Drugs Used in the Last 30 Days Among EFMU and Non-EFMU

	EMFU (n = 42)	Non-EMFU (n = 200)	Sig. (Chi-Square)
Ecstasy	36%	16%	8.62**
Prescription Narcotics	15%	19%	.452
Benzodiazepines	10%	21%	2.96
Heroin	38%	56%	4.46*
Cocaine	29%	39%	1.61
Inhalants	0%	0%	0

*p < .05, ** p < .01

he had been getting high on marijuana laced with embalming fluid mixture. When his stash of the drug dwindled, Billie decided to take a ride with some friends to find his usual drug dealer and purchase a new batch of embalming fluid mixture. Billie drove, and when they got near to where they were going, someone in Billie's car spotted another car nearby which he insisted belonged to members of a rival gang. Billie took off after the car and was able to pull up alongside of it, at which point his friend in the passenger seat fired four shots into the other car. Two of the four occupants of the other car were killed from bullet wounds. After the shooting, however, both cars careened out of control and crashed. Billie survived and was charged with complicity in a homicide. As a defense, he maintained that the embalming fluid mixture that he had been smoking non-stop for two days made him lose his mind temporarily. The court was not convinced and found him guilty. Ultimately the Connecticut Supreme Court affirmed the ruling.

The question of the relationship of embalming fluid mixture use to violence, however, remains an important one and it often is mentioned by clinical treatment providers who work with EFMUs. A computer search by our research team of the last four years of a Connecticut newspaper's archives produced multiple articles about violent incidents in which the police reported perpetrator use of "dust," "illy" or "embalming fluid." Similarly, among members of our sample, 49% of EFMU reported that they tend to start fights or become violent when high compared to 32% of participants who did not report use of embalming fluid mixtures ($p < .04$). As one younger embalming fluid mixture user told us in the in-depth interview component of the study:

> Fighting that is all . . . Fist fighting, where there is pulling hair and everything . . . I don't know because if I am on E [Ecstasy] I am happy. If I do hemey [embalming fluid], I feel evil. My whole face is like . . . guys tell me the whole expression on your face changes. You look evil. And I start trouble. I start looking for trouble.

Another user reported:

> It's a mind-altering drug. If you're mad, you can kill somebody on dust; if you are upset and you're smoking.

Similarly, a third participant noted:

> When they smoke dust, they like to go out and shoot their guns, you know. So they get dusted out and all their problems that they've had they become um . . . more uh, more amped to go and deal with something than they would if they were sober. It almost makes you have like crazy beliefs that you're like someone else, that you have some kind of power, you know.

There was no significant difference between EFMU and non-EFMU in terms of having a history of attempted suicide (about 22% of both groups reported such a history, however, suggesting the importance of regular illicit drug use in a wider set of mental health problems). The non-EFMU in our sample were more likely than EFMU to report a history of receiving mental health treatment (36% vs. 20% respectively, $p < .04$), although this difference may be a function of age differences between the two groups.

Seventeen percent of the embalming fluid mixture users reported suffering from anxiety, while 12% reported depression. Memory problems were cited by 7% of embalming fluid mixture users. For example, one participant who reported he has used the drug off-and-on for 10 years, and in recent years has smoked embalming fluid mixture every day, stated the following:

> Um, my thought process is not as quick as it was, sometimes I find myself stuttering which I never did. . . . 'Cuz I would find myself talking to somebody and I would hear myself [sound effect, stutter] . . . I would stretch words out when I know I never did that before. I would sleep extra late, when I get up from sleeping I would be real stiff 'cuz the embalming fluid in the dust. So, I see some of the things that happen.

Notably, this individual, an African American man who was about 30 years old at the time of the interview, reported that the drug makes it hard for him to fall asleep or to get adequate rest.

EFMU and others in the sample who knew EFMU also reported various bad experiences and bizarre behaviors under the influence of the drug. As one participant noted with reference to people who use embalming fluid mixtures, "I've seen a lot of people walking in the street talking to themselves." Another participant, a non-EFMU in her mid-30s who used a variety of other drugs, commented:

Yeah because sometimes they [EFMU] stay stuck. One time at two o'clock in the morning, there was this guy outside . . . for two hours straight he was like, "Yo, yo, yo, yo . . . where we're going . . . yo, yo, yo, yo. . . ." He stayed like that. I had to give him some milk to bring him down. . . . And I was like, "they put this in dead people and you smoke it?"

One participant described the long-term impact of embalming fluid mixture on her sister-in-law's brother as follows:

My brother's wife; her brother, he didn't know what he was smoking with a couple of friends of him. He went at the top of a building in New York, butt naked and he was thinking that he could fly. And he never came back to himself. . . . He's acting like that . . . he would talk about crazy stuff. . . . Yeah, ever since he did dust . . . Now he does psychiatric medicine and you can get him to do anything you want him to do. They [criminal friends] had him scaling up a building, the window; get into the house to open the door for them . . . And he is like superman scaling up the wall.

A middle-aged female participant who was both a drug user and dealer, described her experience with the drug as well as that of her teenage son in the following way:

I sold it to a few people and then I started smoking some of it. It comes in a little bag–it's very fine. Fine weed . . . yeah, it's weed. It makes maybe a joint and half to two joints. They soak the [weed] in the formaldehyde [and] all kinds of chemicals, and you roll in a joint or smoke it like hash in a pipe. It has a nasty smell. I didn't like the way it made me act . . . I thought someone was chasing me. You smoke a dime [$10] of dust and your head explodes. It is like getting two hits of acid, LSD . . . or whatever. I still don't know if it was real, if I was being chased. It's the kind of high you don't know what's going on and you are so confused and you just want to get straight . . . My son comes here and he had smoked a [dust] joint and he was vomiting, and it was black and there was foam coming from his mouth. He was fifteen.

A number of participants in the study used the term "zombie" to describe regular embalming fluid mixture users. As one man in his mid-20s explained:

> Like I've seen kids smoke so much they can't move . . . they're just zombies. Their eyes are open, and some kids get scared . . . because they are spare time users and you warn them . . . these kids think they're heroes and they hit it as hard as they can and they're laying around . . . and they can't move.

Other study participants, however, discounted the accounts of bizarre behaviors among embalming fluid mixture users. As one such individual stated:

> Yeah, [it's] like an urban myth. My friends do it all the time and they're not going to tell me to do it if it's not okay.

In terms of other health issues, equally high percentages of EFMU and non-EFMU reported being infected with hepatitis C (21% and 25% respectively), with comparatively fewer members of both groups reporting HIV infection (5% and 7% respectively). While 5% of the non-EFMU reported hepatitis B infection, none of the EFMU reported having this disease. About 7% of both groups reported having suffered from an STD. Finally, while 2% of non-EFMU reported suffering from tuberculosis, among the EFMU 7% reported this disease. Additionally, 24% of EFMU reported experiencing a drug overdose, but only one individual indicated that this occurred with embalming fluid mixture.

Finally, beyond health issues, we found that non-EFMU were more likely to report having been incarcerated than EFMU (64% vs. 44% respectively, $p < .03$), although a large percentage of both groups have arrest and incarceration histories. Again, the younger average age of EFMU is likely to account for the fewer number of arrests.

UNCERTAIN CHEMISTRY, DESIRED EFFECTS

Among participants in our sample who were not embalming fluid users–all of whom were heavily involved in other illicit street drug use–only 35% identified embalming fluid as an ingredient in "dust"; and even fewer (31%) reported that it was an ingredient in "wet." While 20% of the non-EFMU believed that PCP was an ingredient in "dust," only 13% reported that it was an ingredient in "wet." Moreover, 54% of non-EFMU stated that they did not know the contents of "dust," while 62% were uncertain of the contents of "wet." As these percentages suggest, while non-users of embalming fluid mixtures generally were aware of the drug, the majority were uncertain about its chemical composition or have their own ideas about its content. As one non-user stated:

Q: So dust . . . what's the composition?
A: Err, I would say, a little rat poison, embalming fluid.
Q: Anything else?
A: Err, I will guess PCP. I am not sure.

Some street drug users, however, were surprised to learn about embalming fluid use from our interview team. As one such individual told us in response to question:

Q: Have you heard of embalming fluid? What is it?
A: They put it in dead people. Hell no. I won't smoke that shit. They put it in dead people. It is being smoked, oh god. It's not funny . . . I want to live. It is being smoked?

High levels of uncertainty–although not to the degree of non-users– also were found among users of embalming fluid mixtures. Among users, 60% reported embalming fluid as an ingredient in "dust," while 50% believed it was an ingredient in "wet." Forty-three percent of EFMU reported that PCP was found in both "dust" and "wet." Finally, while 24% of EFMU said they did not know what "dust" was made of, 36% reported a lack of knowledge concerning the make-up of "wet." Further, the majority (76%) of non-users of embalming fluid mixtures did not know the difference between "dust" and "wet," while 45% of EFMU indicated that they did not know the difference. For example, a participant in the in-depth interviews told us the following:

Q: So what color is it, what does it look like?
A: Black, charcoal black.
Q: What is the composition of black dust? How is it made?
A: To be honest, I don't really know. I just buy it and smoke it. I should know because it's going into my body, but I don't know.
Q: Did you ever ask?
A: No, no. I just smoke it often but not really often. It's not like cocaine [where I] have to know what's in it.

Another embalming fluid mixture user told us:

Q: And what do you think is in the dust?

> A: I heard that it was like rat poison, but I am not really sure. I would obviously want to know since I put it into my body, but I sprinkle it [on marijuana], not like drenched [it] with dust.

In a particularly revealing exchange with a project ethnographer, one individual who had been using embalming fluid mixtures for some time reported the following:

> Q: Tell me just what do you believe is in dust?
> A: I know what's in it. . . . Embalming fluid, which is . . . formaldehyde, right, mint leaves and PCP.
> Q: So there's PCP in it?
> A: Yeah.
> Q: Do you think everyone knows there's PCP in it?
> A: No.
> Q: So did you always know there was PCP in it?
> A: No.
> Q: When did you find out?
> A: It was already too late. I learned that like a year and half ago, two years ago.
> Q: So basically you started smoking without knowing what it was and then just a year ago you found out that it had PCP in it?
> A: Yup.
> Q: So do you know what's PCP?
> A: No, not really.

A number of EFMU reported that they only realized that dust or wet has PCP in it when they underwent urine toxicology following an emergency room visit brought on by drug overdose. As one participant explained:

> I only found out 'cuz one time I had went to the hospital, I was smokin' it and um . . . they had took a urine on me and they said that I was smokin' and it had PCP in it. I didn't even know, until then.

Because of this level of uncertainty, it is not completely clear if drugs sold on the street as "dust," "wet" or "illy" are in fact the same drug, although some users of each of these drugs report embalming fluid is a key ingredient (even if they may be unsure of other contents in the drug they use or of drugs sold under other street names than the one they use).

Also, users described drugs sold with these three street names or even other street names (e.g., tecal, hemmie) as being a dry black powder (dust, illy, tecal) or a wet black powder (wet or wet wet). A long-time embalming fluid user, for example, stated the following:

A: Ah, the first three right there is the same.
Q: Dust, illy and wet, [are] all the same?
A: Yeah, all the same.
Q: Now, some people have also told me that dust comes in a little bag, it's powdery and it's black like you said.
A: Yeah, and wet is like that, too, but it's moist, but it's the same thing. 'Cuz you could make wet into dust in a matter of seconds. All you gotta do is dry it out. Wet is moist and dust is like powdery. Not powdery but it's like dry.
Q: Have you ever tried . . . wet?
A: Yeah. Wet is dust! Yeah it's dust but . . . ok the difference between . . . it's like, ok you've got coffee over here you got dry coffee grinds, then you got wet coffee grinds over here. It's still coffee once you make the coffee right. So you got the dust right here, you got the wet right here. Only difference is this is dry, this is wet.

Complicating the issue of drug content is the fact that embalming fluid mixtures are produced by different drug dealers and it is likely that they use different ingredients and quantities of each ingredient that they combine to produce the final product. Users also mention differences in drug potency, over time and across drug dealers.

LABORATORY FINDINGS

A total of 41 urine samples were collected from participants who reported embalming fluid mixture use during the last 48 hours. Drug testing analysis found that 11 (31%) of these samples tested positive for PCP. This finding provided the first definitive proof that PCP was in fact a component in some, if perhaps not all, embalming fluid mixtures being sold on the streets of Hartford. Additionally, 74% were positive for marijuana, suggesting the widespread practice of combining PCP with marijuana in the preparation of embalming fluid mixtures. Embalming fluid was not detectable with the procedure used in the laboratory testing (given the rapid evaporation of the substance). Notably, 31% of the samples were positive for cocaine, even though some of the participants whose urines were positive for cocaine did not report use of this drug prior to the collection of their urine sample. One interpretation of these findings is that some producers of embalming fluid mixtures lace their product with cocaine unbeknownst to users. Toxicological tests were also performed on the black powder residue still present in 12 drug bags collected by research team members on the streets in areas with significant drug paraphernalia discard (e.g., syringes, water bottles, crack pipes). All of these bags tested positive for PCP.

CONCLUSION: PUBLIC HEALTH IMPLICATIONS

Our laboratory testing confirmed the presence of PCP in at least some of the embalming fluid mixtures sold on the street in Hartford. Moreover, the accounts of EFMU and other drug users who interact with them confirm drug-related experiences and behaviors that parallel descriptions in the PCP literature (e.g., acting like a "zombie," getting "stuck," exhibiting an increased propensity for acts of violence). These findings affirm that we are in the midst of what may be a significant new wave of PCP use, especially among young drug users in the inner city.

While we were not able to test for the presence of embalming fluid in either the urine samples of participants or in the small plastic bags that had been used to hold the drug, participants' descriptions of the smell exuded by the drug match the quite distinct odor of formaldehyde, suggesting the likelihood that embalming fluid is in fact also an ingredient in the dry or wet black powder drug mixtures sold on the street as "dust," "wet" or by other names. While it is unclear if there are health risks associated with smoking formaldehyde, as the substance may be destroyed during the burning process, there are definite risks associated with overexposure to or consumption of liquid formaldehyde including coma, bodily weakness, roaring in the ears, dizziness, convulsions, kidney damage, and possible death (Hawkins et al., 1994; Schulz et al., 1988).

Additionally, our laboratory testing suggested that in at least some batches of embalming fluid mixture, cocaine may be a component. Definitive testing of actual drug samples from a range of dealers and in different forms (i.e., wet and dry), however, is needed to confirm the range of ingredients that are poured into embalming fluid mixtures and consumed by users. The co-presence of cocaine, an addictive drug and a strong central nervous system stimulant (and a drug known to damage the functioning of the immune system) and PCP, a tranquilizer, would make embalming fluid mixtures particularly potent substances, especially for newer users with limited experience with such powerful psychotropic chemicals.

As has been stressed, our study also found that users of embalming fluid mixtures are often quite unsure about the contents of the drug. While a certain degree of uncertainty about drug content is not unusual among illicit users, and has certainly been quite widely reported for other drugs such as ecstasy or with reference to the substances that are used to "cut" (dilute) drugs like heroin (Singer, in press), confusion or vagueness about content seems to be particularly acute among users of embalming fluid mixtures. While some users either assume or suspect the presence of PCP in the drug, others are unaware of the presence of this potent tranquilizer in the drug. Moreover, knowing that a substance called PCP is in embalming fluid mixture does not mean that users have much knowledge of PCP. Similarly, while most users are aware that embalming fluid is in the drug, this is not the case with all users. Finally, very few of the EFMU in our sample expressed the belief that cocaine may be an ingredient, although its presence in at least some of "dust" or "wet" sold on the street was suggested by our laboratory findings. (Of course, those individuals who were tested and found to be positive for cocaine may have used the drug separately from their use of embalming fluid mixture and misreported this use to us at the time of testing; this is unlikely, however, given the fact that they tended to be forthcoming about other drugs they had consumed prior to the analysis.)

The findings of this study are of particular concern from a public health perspective. As noted, embalming fluid mixture users tend to be young. Although we did not interview individuals below the age of 18, participants reported to us that the drug is being used by inner city teens who fall below this age. Additionally, we found that EFMU are polydrug users and are also consuming a range of other potent drugs as well. In other words, on top of the already existing inner city drug crisis, a new wave of PCP mixed with other substances is finding a significant market among inner city youth and young adults, as well as slowly making its way into the drug repertoires of middle-aged illicit drug users. The arrival of this wave of PCP use comes at a time when other new drugs, such as ecstasy and prescription pain killers, are also becoming ever more widely used in the inner city. While many older, experienced drug users are well-versed about possible drug contents and the regulation and management of their illicit drug doses (although never with precise control as indicated by the frequency of drug overdosing), younger, less experienced drug users, especially those who are unaware of possible drug content, may be particularly vulnerable to harmful illicit drug experiences (e.g., by unwittingly mixing PCP-containing embalming fluid mixture with other central nervous system depressants like alcohol or heroin). While of an anecdotal nature, our participants described a number of examples of health deficits among embalming fluid mixture users whom they know as well as their own bad experiences with the drug.

In our own assessment of the local public health and drug treatment system, awareness of the presence of a significant wave of PCP use appears to be quite limited. For example, members of our research team recently participated in a citywide meeting of drug treatment providers, community-based organizations, the police department, and service providers organized by the Hartford Department of Health and Social Services, to discuss changing trends of drug use in the city and available organizational strengths and resources for responding to the health and social consequences of these changes. While participants produced a list of changes in local drug use patterns (e.g., the spread of ecstasy to street drug users, illicit use of pharmaceutical drugs, the growing prevalence of drug mixing), and while there was a strong focus among changing drug use patterns among youth in the inner city, PCP was not mentioned by any of the participants (except members of our research team). Notably, the representative of the Hartford Police Department stated that the only new drug he was aware of that was being sold on the street was Viagra.

Finally, our whole sample of not-in-treatment active drug users suffers from a considerable infectious disease burden compared to the general U.S. population, making them a group of concern for the public health system. Beyond this general pattern, differences are evident in the morbidity profiles of EFMU and non-EFMU that merit closer public health attention in terms of disease control.

In sum, the findings of our study suggest the critical importance of local sites maintaining systems for the identification and tracking of emergent and changing drug use patterns across the full range–by age, ethnicity, social class and other characteristics–of drug users (Agar and Reisinger, 1999; Siegal et al., 2000; Singer et al., in press(b)). Drug use patterns are not stagnant; rather they are in constant flux in response to a range of factors from the War on Drugs to the introduction of new pharmaceutical products with potential psychotropic effects. Additionally, to be effective, drug monitoring systems need to be linked and closely coordinated with local public health officials and drug treatment providers, the local school system, hospitals and clinics, and community organizations, to allow the rapid movement of research findings to individuals and institutions responsible for protecting the health and well-being of the community. Given the noted infectious disease burden of illicit drug-using populations, the building of partnerships between drug researchers and service and treatment providers who serve drug-using populations should be a central item on local public health agendas. While our findings on the chemical content of embalming fluid mixtures and the reports of users and their associates are suggestive, further research is needed to definitively identify the chemical composition of this drug, as well as to assess the longer-term health and social consequences of its use over time, especially among inner city populations already at high risk from a range of health threats.

REFERENCES

Agar, M. & Reisinger, H. S. (1999). Numbers and patterns: Heroin indicators and what they represent. *Human Organization* 58 (4): 365-374.

Elwood, W. (1998). *"Fry": A Study of Adolescents' Use of Embalming Fluid with Marijuana and Tobacco.* Austin, TX: Texas Commission on Alcohol and Drugs.

Farber, N. & Olney, J. (2003). Drugs of abuse that cause developing neurons to commit suicide. *Brain Research and Developmental Brain Research* 147 (1-2): 37-45.

Hawkins, K., Schwartz-Thompson, J. & Kahane, A. (1994). Abuse of formaldehyde-laced marijuana may cause dysmensia. *Journal of Neuropsychiatry and Clinical Neurosciences* 6: 67.

Hoaken, P. & Stewart, S. (2003). Drugs of abuse and the elicitation of human aggressive behavior. *Addictive Behavior* 28 (9): 1533-1554.

Holland, J., Nelson, L., Ravikumar, R. & Elwood, W. (1998). Embalming fluid-soaked marijuana: New high or new guise for PCP? *Journal of Psychoactive Drugs* 30 (2): 215-219.

James, W. & Johnson, S. (1996). *Doin' Drugs: Patterns of African American Addiction.* Austin: University of Texas Press.

Lerner, S. E. & Burns, R. S. (1978). Phencyclidine use among youth: History, epidemiology, and acute and chronic intoxication. In *NIDA Research Monograph, Phencyclidine (PCP) Abuse: An Appraisal* No. 21: 66-118.

Mokhlesi, B., Garimella, P., Joffe, A., & Velho, V. (2004). Street drug abuse leading to critical illness. *Intensive Care Medicine* 1, 45-56.

National Household Survey on Drug Abuse (1979). *Main Findings.* Washington, DC: U.S. Department of Health and Human Services.

Peters, R. C. & Stillman, R. C. (1978). Phencyclidine: An overview. In *NIDA Research Monograph, Phencyclidine (PCP) Abuse: An Appraisal* No. 21: 1-17.

Shulz, P. J., Jones, J. & Pattern, B. (1988). Encephalopathy and rhabdomyolysis from ingesting formaldehyde dipped cigarettes [Abstract]. *Neurology* 38 (Supplement 1): 297.

Siegal, H., Carlson, R., Kenne, D., Starr, S. & Stephens, R. (2000). The Ohio Substance Abuse Monitoring Network: Constructing and operating a statewide epidemiologic intelligence system. *American Journal of Public Health* 90 (12): 1835-7.

Singer, M. (2006). *Something Dangerous: Emergent and Changing Illicit Drug Use and Community Health.* Prospect Heights, IL: Waveland Press.

Singer, M., Clair, S., Schensul, J., Huebner, C., Eiserman, J., Pino, R. & Garcia, J. (in press (a)). Dust in the wind: The growing use of embalming fluid among youth in Hartford, CT. *Substance Use and Misuse.*

Singer, M., Juvalis, J. A. & Weeks, M. (2000). High on illy: Studying an emergent drug problem in Hartford, CT. *Medical Anthropology* 18: 365-388.

Singer, M., Stopka, T., Shaw, S., Santilices, C., Buchanan, D., Teng, W., Khoshnood, K. & Heimer, R. (in press (b)). Lessons from the field: From research to application in the fight against AIDS among injection drug users in three New England cities. *Human Organization.*

Singer, M., Stopka, T., Siano, C., Springer, K., Barton, G., Khoshnood, K., Gorry de Puga, A. & Heimer, R. (2000). The social geography of AIDS and hepatitis risk: Qualitative approaches for assessing local differences in sterile syringe access among injection drug users. *American Journal of Public Health* 90 (7): 1049-1056.

Spector, I. (1985). AMP: A new form of marijuana. *Journal of Clinical Psychiatry* 46: 498-499.

Wish, E. D. (1986). PCP and crime: Just another illicit drug? In *NIDA Research Monograph, Number 64, Phencyclidine: An Update*: 174-189.

Under the Counter:
The Diffusion of Narcotic Analgesics
to the Inner City Street

James Vivian, PhD
Hassan Saleheen, MD
Merrill Singer, PhD
Juhem Navarro, MA
Greg Mirhej, MA

SUMMARY. During the past decade, there has been a well-documented rise in the non-medical use of prescription painkillers, often referred to as narcotics analgesics (NA). Relatively little is known, however, about who these users are, the range of health and social consequences associated with their use, and the presence of illicit NA use on the inner city street. Results of a survey conducted with a sample of 242 street drug users indicated that NA use is now widespread in the inner

Dr. James Vivian is Chief Data Analyst at the Hispanic Health Council.

Dr. Hassan Saleheen is Data Analyst on the Building Community Responses project.

Dr. Merrill Singer is Director of the Center for Community Health Research of the Hispanic Health Council and Principal Investigator on the CDC-funded Building Community Responses to Risks of Emergent Drug Use project.

Juhem Navarro is Data Manager on the Building Community Responses project.

Greg Mirhej is Project Coordinator of the Building Community Responses project.

Address correspondence to: James Vivian, PhD, Hispanic Health Council, 175 Main Street, Hartford, CT 06106 (E-mail: jimv@hispanichealth.com).

[Haworth co-indexing entry note]: "Under the Counter: The Diffusion of Narcotic Analgesics to the Inner City Street." Vivian, James et al. Co-published simultaneously in *Journal of Ethnicity in Substance Abuse* (The Haworth Press, Inc.) Vol. 4, No. 2, 2005, pp. 97-114; and: *New Drugs on the Street: Changing Inner City Patterns of Illicit Consumption* (ed: Merrill Singer) The Haworth Press, Inc., 2005, pp. 97-114. Single or multiple copies of this article are available for a fee from The Haworth Document Delivery Service [1-800- HAWORTH, 9:00 a.m. - 5:00 p.m. (EST). E-mail address: docdelivery@haworthpress.com].

Available online at http://www.haworthpress.com/web/JESA
doi:10.1300/J233v04n02_05

city, and that it is associated with a number of serious health and psychiatric conditions. Other characteristics of this emerging drug user group are explored and the need for future research is highlighted. *[Article copies available for a fee from The Haworth Document Delivery Service: 1-800-HAWORTH. E-mail address: <docdelivery@haworthpress.com> Website: <http://www.HaworthPress.com> © 2005 by The Haworth Press, Inc. All rights reserved.]*

KEYWORDS. Narcotic analgesics, substance abuse

This paper reports findings from an ongoing, CDC-funded investigation of emergent patterns of drug abuse among city drug users in Hartford, Connecticut. The study reported here was designed to examine the presence of illicit use of Narcotic Analgesics (NA) in the inner city, factors associated with NA use in this context, and the impact of NA use on the health and social well-being of low-income, vulnerable populations with disproportionate drug-related health and other health issues. The goal of this investigation is the development of insights for use in the creation of evidence-based intervention approaches with inner city NA users. A focus on outreach-recruited populations that are omitted from many of the primary sources of data on drug abuse provides needed public health information on inner city NA use and its consequences for communities, treatment providers and policymakers.

RISING RATES OF NA USE

The problem of non-medical use of prescription drugs has become enormous in recent years. It is estimated, for example, that over 10% of the U.S. population over the age of 12 engaged in this practice at least once during 2003 (National Survey on Drug Use and Health, 2004). Painkillers, or Narcotic Analgesics, are the most commonly abused prescription drugs and are now second only to marijuana as the nation's most abused drug (Janofsky, 2004). Marketed under brand names like Vicodin (hydrocodone), OxyContin (oxycodone), Percocet (also contains oxycodone), Demerol (meperidine) and Darvon (propoxyphene), these drugs all fall under the opiate classification and are thus capable of providing symptom-relief from pain. In large enough doses, NAs can also produce a euphoric effect analogous to that produced by other well-known and commonly abused natural opiates like heroin. And like heroin, NAs are habit-forming when taken for extended periods of time.

From 1994 to 2001, according to Drug Abuse Warning Network (DAWN), there was a 117% increase in Emergency Department (ED) mentions related to NA abuse (The DAWN Report, 2003). While this rising trend in NA abuse is found for virtually all types of NAs (except codeine), the largest increases in ED mentions are found for oxycodone (352%), methadone (230%), morphine (210%) and hydrocodone (131%). OxyContin diversion and abuse has been of particular concern to both law enforcement and health care professionals. ED mentions for single-entity oxycodone (only drug involved) since the release of Oxycontin (a controlled release form of the schedule II narcotic) have increased from as few as 100 in 1996 to 14,996 in 2002, an upsurge more dramatic than is found in all other NAs combined (DEA, 2003). Ethnographic reports emanating from the Community Epidemiology Work Group (CEWG) indicate that oxycodone and hydrocodone, in particular, are increasing in popularity among traditional drug-abusing populations in major urban centers like St. Louis, Denver, San Francisco, Baltimore, Philadelphia and in Phoenix, where the ED rate for NAs exceeded the rate for all other drugs (CEWG, 6/2003). Notably, in several other cities, ED rates for NAs exceeded rates for heroin mentions.

Treatment admission rates for abuse of narcotic painkillers more than doubled between 1992 and 2000. This increase was considerably larger for NAs (76%) than for treatment admissions generally (9%) and primary heroin treatment admissions (16%) between 1997 and 2000 (The DASIS Report, 2003). This rise can be explained, in part, by the substantial increase in the proportion of new users of NAs (those entering treatment within three years of initiating use) during this same period (30% in 1997, 41% in 2000). Perhaps the most disturbing trend of all is the fact that the recent rise in the prevalence of nonmedical NA use is found among adolescents and young adults. According to National Household Survey on Drug Abuse (2003), the initiation of prescription drug abuse occurs primarily among people aged 12 to 25, and new use of prescription pain relievers (NAs) shows the sharpest rise, from about 400,000 in the mid-80s to over 2 million in 2000.

ILLICIT NA USERS

Little is known about habitual or recreational users of NAs. The demographic information provided in the aforementioned national reports provides only a limited amount of data. The DAWN (Drug Abuse Warning Network) report, for example, informs us that the average age of NA abusers visiting an ED was 37, with rates peaking in the 26 to 34 age group (69 per 100,000 population). For both men and women, hydrocodone and oxycodone were most frequently mentioned among the NAs and overall ED rates were slightly, though not substantially, higher for men than for women. In 2001, the majority of ED patients who reported NA abuse were white (62,937) while 9,986 were black and 8,329 Hispanic, proportions relative to their numbers in the population. For each racial/ethnic group, the most frequently named NAs were hydrocodone, oxycodone and methadone. Finally, the DAWN report goes on to show that the majority of ED mentions for NA abuse involved more than one drug (72%). The most frequently named substance used in conjunction with NAs was cocaine though substantial numbers also mention benzodiazepines and alcohol. The picture that thus emerges from these data is of a white, poly-substance abusing 30-something adult whose NA of choice is either hydrocodone (i.e., Vicodin) or oxycodone (i.e., OxyContin).

More detailed demographic and related information was recently provided by Miller and Greenfield (2004) who examined characteristics of hydrocodone and oxycodone dependence in an addiction treatment population. Patients in their sample were more likely to be younger, female, white, have other medical diagnoses and have a history of pain management therapy. And because the NA users in the study were also more likely to test positive for virtually every drug (except marijuana) than their non-NA user counterparts, the authors reasonably conclude that a history of (any) substance abuse can be taken as a risk factor for NA abuse in particular. It should be noted, however, that the setting for this study was a small, private inpatient facility in the Midwest. As such, the fact that the sample was predominantly white, middle-class, and suburban or rural residents with private insurance comes as no surprise.

Findings like these might lead to the conclusion (as have many newspaper reports) that NA abuse is not common among low-income ethnic/minority groups. Such a conclusion is unwarranted and shortsighted. In the first place, non-representative samples of the kind described above cannot serve as the basis for our understanding of NA or any other kind of substance abuse. It goes without saying that while there are significantly fewer black and Hispanic NA abusers overall, reported numbers do not appear to be out of proportion to their numbers in the overall population. Also, there is reason to believe that NHSDA and DAWN data underestimate, perhaps dramatically, the prevalence of NA use among traditional inner city drug-using populations who are less likely to be included in household surveys or to avail themselves of emergency services in hospitals. So, while the reports mentioned above give us a useful overview of the dramatic rise in NA abuse nationwide, considerably more focus should be placed on understanding the demographic and other characteristics of this growing population.

The most comprehensive analysis of demographic factors associated with prescription drug abuse in general, and NA abuse in particular, was recently provided by Simoni-Wastila and her colleagues (Simoni-Wastila, Ritter, and Strickler, 2004; Simoni-Wastila and Strickler, 2004). Using logistic regression with NHSDA data, these authors report in one study that significant risk factors for "problem" NA abuse (i.e., DSM-dependence) included being female and unmarried (Simoni-Wastila and Strickler, 2004), while in another study, risk factors for non-medical NA use more generally (i.e., not necessarily "problem" use according to the authors) included being white, female, in poor health and daily alcohol or illicit drug use (Simoni-Wastila, Ritter, and Strickler, 2004). Marital status, income and having health insurance did not distinguish between NA users and non-users in the latter study. It is worth noting that in the former study, where the outcome was based on DSM criteria for heavy use and dependence, factors commonly expected to be associated with NA abuse were not associated (e.g., ethnicity, suburban vs. urban residence, education, income).

Health/Mortality Risks of Illicit NA Use

Recent studies have found both an alarming number of deaths associated with NA abuse in general and their combined use with benzodiazepines and other opiates in particular (U.S. Dept. of Justice report, 2002; Cone et al., 2003). DAWN reports, for example, that the number of oxycodone-related deaths more than quadrupled from 1996 to 1999. The CEWG further indicates that the number of NA-related death mentions exceeded those for cocaine, heroin/morphine, marijuana and methamphetamine in 11 of 20 cities included in the DAWN mortality system (CEWG, 2003). Cone et al. (2003) constructed an oxycodone postmortem database from cases solicited from Medical Examiner/Coroner offices in 23 states from August, 1999 through mid-January, 2002. The vast majority of cases were described as "multiple drug abuse deaths" in which there was at least one other plausible contributory drug in addition to oxycodone. The most prevalent drug combinations, in order of frequency of mentions, were oxycodone used with diazepam (valium), hydrocodone (e.g., Vicodin), alcohol, and cocaine with less prevalence of benzodiazepines, opiates and antidepressants.

PURPOSE OF STUDY

The primary purpose of the present study, which was part of a larger Centers for Disease Control and Prevention (CDC)-funded investigation of emergent and changing drug use patterns (Singer and Mirhej, 2004), was to investigate the extent to which prescription narcotics have diffused "to the street" in order to better assist health care providers who work with this vulnerable population in the development of needed public health responses. In addition to rates of use across demographic groupings, we also explore the association between NA use and various health consequences. We pay particular attention to the relationship between NA use and drug overdose. To this end, we obtained mortality data from the state of Connecticut Medical Examiner's office as another indication of the use and consequences of NAs in this particular geographical locale.

Methods

Sample Selection/Recruitment

The study was carried out in Hartford, CT, a city whose population is currently estimated to be just under 130,000. The city is ethnically diverse (38.1% African American, 40.5% Hispanic/Puerto Rican, 27.7% white), and generally impoverished (i.e., estimated to be the fourth poorest moderate-sized U.S. city), with high rates of unemployment, violence, drug abuse and AIDS cases (Himmelgreen and Singer, 1998).

Because our intention was to target not-in-treatment drug users, sample participants were recruited in areas of the city known from past studies to have comparatively high concentrations of drug-related activities. To recruit a study sample that reasonably reflects the street drug-using population, sampling was thus based on a neighborhood sampling design. Outreach workers who matched the target sample by gender, language and ethnicity frequented these areas and approached men and women they encountered on the street. Conversations typically began with a brief description of the project. Potential participants were then asked a brief set of questions to determine their eligibility for the study. Eligible participants had to be over 18 years of age, reported recent (i.e., 30 days) use of drugs other than alcohol and marijuana, and had not been in drug treatment (including detox, self-help programs) during the last 30 days. Candidates could be excluded from participation if project staff determined that they did not clearly understand the consent process or if they made verbal threats or became violent (although there were no exclusions on these grounds). Media advertisement was also used to help attract participants, especially those who tend to be underrepresented in surveys of active drug users (i.e., 18-25 year olds). Interested, eligible subjects were given an appointment at The Hispanic Health Council offices in Hartford where they were led through the formal consent process, interviewed for approximately one hour and, where appropriate, referred to agency or other community-based service providers. A final sample (n = 242) of drug users was thus obtained.

Measures

The survey instrument used in this project was based on the AIDS Risk Assessment (ARA) developed originally by Mark Williams for use with drug users in Houston (Joe and Simpson, 1993). The ARA systematically collects information on drug use, syringe-related and sex-related AIDS risk behaviors, health status, and related health information. To provide measures of a broad range of outcomes and risk behaviors, we adapted the instrument to provide information concerning drug use (recent use of NAs–Methadone, OxyContin, Percocet, Vicodin–injection drug use, Marijuana, Crack, Heroin, Benzodiazepines, Club Drugs), health status (Hepatitis B, Hepatitis C, STD, drug overdose and HIV), psychiatric conditions, treatment history and sexual risk behavior.

RESULTS

Study Participants

A total of 242 individuals participated in the study. Ranging in age from 18-57 (Mean age = 33.15/Median = 33.0/SD = 9.93), the sample reflected the ethnic composition of the city of Hartford with approximately 1/3 identified as black/African American (34.5%), 1/5 white (21.2%), and almost 1/2 Latino/Puerto Rican (44.2%). These figures roughly correspond to recent U.S. Census data for the city of Hartford in 2000. The sample was predominantly male (61.6%) but with a sizeable percentage of female participants (38.4%).

Overall Rates of NA Use

As seen in Table 1, over 1/2 of the sample (51.7%) reported illicit use of NAs at some point in their lives with more than 1/5 (21.5%) using

TABLE 1. Rates of Narcotic Analgesic Use in Study Sample (n = 242)

Drug	Ever Used N (%)	Used in past 30 days N (%)
OxyContin	41 (16.9)	14 (5.8)
Other Oxycodone (i.e., Percodan/Percocet)	78 (32.2)	31 (12.8)
Hydrocodone (Vicodin)	21 (8.7)	7 (2.9)
Methadone	78 (32.2)	20 (8.3)
Overall NA use	125 (51.7)	52 (21.5)

within the past 30 days. Oxycodone (Percocet) and methadone were the most likely of the NAs to have been tried, but Oxycodone in the form of Percocet was the most widely used recently (12.8%).

Demographic Comparison of NA Users and Non-Users

As indicated in Table 2, NA users (i.e., those using in past 30 days) did not differ from non-users in terms of age and gender. Significant demographic differences were noted, however, in the ethnic and educational background of users and non-users. Specifically, it appears that white participants were significantly more likely to have used NAs recently (39.6% of white participants) than either black (15.4%) or Latino/Puerto Rican (17.0%) participants. Further, a relationship between educational attainment and NA use is indicated by the fact that 29.4% of those with at least a high school degree reported recent NA use compared to 15.9% of those with less education.

Patterns of (Other) Drug Use Among NA Users

Active NA users and non-users did not differ in their use of many other drugs including PCP, crack, cocaine, heroin club drugs and amphetamines (see Table 3). Overall, NA users were not any more likely to

TABLE 2. Demographic Comparison of Active NA Users and Non-Users (N = 242).

	Active NA User n = 52 (21.5%)	Non-user n = 190 (78.5%)	Sig.
Age	Mean = 34.65	Mean = 35.00	n.s.
Age categories	N (% of users)	N (% of non-users)	n.s
18-25	12 (23.5)	69 (36.5)	
26-30	7 (13.7)	17 (9.0)	
31-40	17 (33.3)	56 (29.6)	
41+	15 (29.4)	47 (24.9)	
Gender			n.s.
Male	29 (55.8)	120 (63.2)	
Female	23 (44.2)	70 (36.8)	
Ethnicity			p < .006
Black	12 (23.5)	66 (35.3)	
White	19 (37.3)	29 (15.5)	
Puerto-Rican	17 (33.3)	83 (44.4)	
Other	3 (5.9)	9 (4.8)	
Educational level			p < .04
Less than HS diploma	20 (40.0)	106 (56.4)	
HS diploma or beyond	30 (60.0)	82 (43.6)	

inject drugs than non-users, though a difference was obtained on lique-fied crack injection specifically. Though the numbers were relatively small in each case, it appears that a higher percentage of NA users (11.5%) injected crack in the previous month than non-users (1.6%). NA users were also more likely to use benzodiazepines (48.1%) than non-users (11.1%), suggesting that prescription drugs in general are more widely abused by this group. A near significant difference was

TABLE 3. Recent Drug Use Trends Among Active NA Users and Non-Users

Drug	Active NA User (n = 52)	Non-user (n = 190)
Marijuana* .003	24 (46.2)	130 (68.4)
Dust/PCP	7 (13.5)	35 (18.4)
Crack	34 (65.4)	112 (58.9)
Cocaine	8 (15.4)	38 (20.0)
Heroin (oral/nasal)	18 (34.6)	61 (32.1)
Injection Drug Use	21 (40.4)	62 (32.6)
–inject crack* (.001)	6 (11.5)	3 (1.6)
–inject cocaine	11 (21.2)	49 (25.8)
–inject heroin	18 (34.6)	61 (32.1)
Benzodiazepines** (.0001)	25 (48.1)	21 (11.1)
Club Drugs	10 (19.2)	41 (21.6)
Crystal Meth* (.06)	1 (1.9)	0 (0.0)
Amphetamines	0 (0.0)	0 (0.0)

also obtained on recent use of crystal meth (p < .06) though it should be pointed out that there was only a single case of recent use of this drug overall. Recent use of marijuana was more commonly reported among non-users of NAs (68.4%) than among users (46.2%).

Friends' Use of Drugs

Participants also were asked to indicate how many of their friends used different types of drugs during the past month. In no case did non-users of NAs report higher rates of friends' drug use than NA users. Users, however, were more likely to report that most/all of their friends used prescription drugs during this time period (44.2%) than non-users (15.8%). In addition, users reported significantly higher rates of crystal meth (16.3% vs. 4.4%) and ketamine (6.1% vs. 0.5%) than non-users though these rates were relatively low overall.

Treatment History

As seen in Table 4, almost 3/4 of NA users in our sample reported having been in detox at some point in their lives (73.1%) and just over 1/2 have been in long-term, inpatient rehab (52.9%). A majority also reported having received mental health treatment (51.9%). These rates are significantly higher than those reported by non-users of NAs for detox (56.6%), long-term rehab (31.4%) and mental health treatment (28.2%).

Health/Psychiatric Problems of NA Users and Non-Users

NA use was found to be associated with a range of undesirable health and psychiatric conditions. As depicted in Table 5, rates of Hepatitis C and liver disease more generally were significantly higher among NA users (36.5%, 11.5%) than among non-users (20.5%, 2.6%). Because injection drug use was slightly, though not significantly, higher among NA users (see Table 3), one might conclude that these higher rates of Hepatitis C, in particular, derive from injection drug use. To tease apart the relative influence of NA use and injection drug use on Hepatitis C, a logistic regression analysis was performed with Hepatitis status as the

TABLE 4. Treatment History of NA Users and Non-Users

Treatment type	Active NA User (n = 52)	Non-user (190)
Ever been in detox* (p < .03)	38 (73.1)	107 (56.6)
Ever been in rehab* (p < .004)	27 (52.9)	59 (31.4)
Ever received mental health treatment* (p < .001)	27 (51.9)	53 (28.2)

TABLE 5. Health Problems of NA Users and Non-Users.

Health problem	Active NA User (n = 52)	Non-user (190)
Hepatitis C (p < .02)	19 (36.5)	39 (20.5)
Liver Disease (p < .02)	6 (11.5)	5 (2.6)
Seizures (p < .03)	5 (9.6)	5 (2.6)
Memory problem (p < .008)	9 (17.3)	11 (5.8)
Anxiety (p < .04)	12 (23.5)	23 (12.2)
Anxiety disorder (p < .04)	18 (34.6)	39 (20.9)
Worsened mental illness (p < .05)	9 (17.3)	15 (7.9)
Difficulty breathing (p < .04)	6 (11.8)	8 (4.3)
Ever had drug overdose (p < .04)	18 (34.6)	40 (21.1)
Among those with history of overdose	18	40
# times overdosed (p < .04)		
–once	1 (5.6)	15 (38.5)
–twice	5 (27.8)	6 (15.4)
–3 or more times	12 (66.7)	18 (46.2)

dichotomous outcome measure and recent NA use and injection drug use as categorical predictors. Age, ethnicity and gender were also entered as demographic covariates. Not surprisingly, the overall model was significant (Chi-square(5) = 77.95; p < .0001) and correctly classified 81.3% of cases in terms of Hepatitis C status. Interestingly, both injected drugs and recent NA use (but none of the demographic controls) were independently associated with Hepatitis C status in the overall adjusted model. While the effect appears to be stronger for drug injection (Odds Ratio = 16.81; 95% CI = 7.53-37.52), the effect is nevertheless notable for recent NA use (Odds Ratio = 3.23; 95% CI = 1.34-7.78), indicating that recent NA users were over three times more likely (223%) than non-users to have Hepatitis C.

Results in Table 5 also show that NA users were significantly more likely to report a history of seizures, memory problems, difficulty breathing and drug overdose than non-users. With respect to drug overdose, NA users were not only more likely than non-users to have had this painful experience, but to have had it multiple times.

Of the various psychiatric conditions considered, NA use appears to be associated with anxiety in particular. As Table 5 indicates, proportionately more NA users reported a history of anxiety (23.5%) than nonusers (12.2%). Further supporting the link between NA use and psychiatric comorbidity, it should be pointed out that NA users were also significantly more likely than non-users to claim that their drug use "caused" an anxiety disorder (34.6% vs. 20.9%) and that it "worsened their mental illness" (17.3% vs. 7.9%).

Mortality Associated with NA Use

To further assess the consequences of NA use, we moved beyond our own data set and analyzed data from the state of Connecticut Medical Examiner's office for the years 1997 to 2002 (see Tables 6 and 7). Specifically, we identified the total number of drug-related deaths and the number of deaths where a Narcotic Analgesic was identified in post-mortem blood tests. NAs identified in the Medical Examiner data included methadone, oxycodone, hydrocodone, codeine, fentanyl, hydromorphone, meperidine, petazocine, and propoxyphene.

Overall, NAs were identified in 15.2% of the drug-related deaths in the state of Connecticut between 1997 and 2002, making it the fourth category of drug most frequently associated with mortality (following heroin/morphine, alcohol, and cocaine). Mirroring the rising trend in NA use nationwide, NA-associated mortality for the entire state of Connecticut rose considerably from a low of 10.6% of the cases in 1999 to 24.0% of the cases in 2002. This trend also was noted in the city of Hartford, specifically, where the lowest (1.6%) and highest (21.4%) rates of NA-associated mortality were similarly found in 1999 and 2002, respectively.

TABLE 6. Mortality Associated with NA Use in State of Connecticut (1997-2002)

Year	Overall N	NA-deaths	% (of total drug-related deaths)
1997	384	52	13.5
1998	408	50	12.3
1999	454	48	10.6
2000	524	74	14.1
2001	449	75	16.7
2002	425	102	24.0
Overall	2644	401	15.2

TABLE 7. Mortality Associated with NA Use in Hartford, CT (1997-2002)

Year	Overall N	NA-deaths	% (of total drug-related deaths)
1997	48	6	12.5
1998	38	2	5.3
1999	61	1	1.6
2000	71	7	9.9
2001	58	11	19.0
2002	28	6	21.4
Overall	304	33	10.92

DISCUSSION

The central questions underlying the present investigation concerned the degree to which illicit NA use has diffused to the inner city street and the characteristics of this emerging drug-using population. With respect to diffusion, it is clear from the present results that NA use is widespread in the inner city among both men and women of varying ages. With respect to ethnic identity, it appears that whites in the inner city are somewhat more likely to abuse NAs than other ethnic groups. So, while the diffusion of NAs to the inner city is not restricted to whites, it remains to be seen whether the growing trend in NA use nationwide will spread to other ethnic groups in significant numbers.

Results also highlighted some other characteristics of this drug-using group. Of particular note is the fact that NA users were more likely than non-users to abuse Benzodiazepines and to associate with people who also abuse prescription drugs. These findings are notable for a couple of reasons. In the first place, opiate/benzodiazepine combinations are particularly dangerous and thus put users at increased risk for overdose (e.g., Iguchi, Handelsman, Bickel, and Griffiths, 1993; Darke, Ross, Zador, and Sunjic, 2000). This might at least partially explain the fact that NA users in the present study were significantly more likely to report drug-related overdose than non-users. Additionally, the fact that NA users associate with others who abuse prescription drugs suggests that there may be social networks of people in the inner city that are drawn to the abuse of prescription drugs more generally. It will be important to learn more about this emerging user group and their drug use histories.

The subsample of participants who reported using NAs in the past 30 days (n = 52) were asked additional questions that were intended to provide us with further insight into characteristics of the inner city NA user. While some of the participants reported using NAs for several years, the majority of participants in our sample (61%) are recent initiates, having used for one year or less. But while their use has not been longstanding, a sizeable percentage of our sample reported what might be considered fairly intense or regular use of NAs following initiation (70% use daily or several times per week). Further supporting the notion that NAs have diffused to the street, the most frequently mentioned source of NAs (58%) were street drug dealers and almost one-half (43%) indicated that they have sold prescription drugs themselves.

What leads one to abuse NAs? Because these drugs can be legally prescribed, it is not surprising that early reports identified chronic pain and post-surgical complications as potential pathways to abuse. It remains to be seen, however, whether the majority of individuals who abuse NAs do so (at least initially) to manage pain, to deal with emotional distress or simply to get high. The little data that are available in this regard suggest either that NA abuse is typically precipitated by either the legitimate need for pain relief (i.e., post-accident/surgical complications–Cone et al., 2004), a state of general ill-health (Simoni-Wastila, Ritter, and Strickler, 2004) or, in other cases, as a substitute opiate for heroin among longer-term addicts who are unable to obtain the latter drug (Ohio Substance Abuse Monitoring Network, 2003). Some insight into the motivation to use NAs was offered by The Ohio Substance Abuse Monitoring Network (OSAM) which recently identified three types of NA abusers (OSAM, 2003). One group consisted of daily users who considered NAs their primary drug of choice. Another group consisted of primary heroin users who substituted NAs as needed. A third group, which used NAs occasionally, typically combined them with other substances. It may be the case, therefore, that motivation for NA use varies depending on the user's medical and drug history, current drug use, and availability of NAs more generally.

Though motivations for use were not explored directly in the present study, some inferences might be drawn from findings concerning increased psychiatric symptomatology among NA users. The fact that NA users were significantly more likely to report a range of symptoms from memory problems and difficulty breathing to anxiety and anxiety disorders suggests that underlying psychiatric morbidity may have predisposed them to abuse NAs. The attraction that NAs hold for some people might thus be the symptom relief they provide for emotionally vulnerable individuals. Such an interpretation is, of course, tentative given the correlational nature of the data. It is possible, for example, that NA abuse precipitates a psychiatric condition rather than the other way around.

Perhaps the most disturbing trend in the data concerns the association between NA abuse and Hepatitis C (Table 5). The fact that NA users were over three times as likely to be diagnosed with this devastating illness than non-users, combined with the fact that this effect remains even after controlling for injection drug use, suggests that illicit use of NAs may represent an important factor in the spread of Hepatitis C. The mechanism underlying this relationship, however, remains unclear and warrants further investigation.

CONCLUSION

It is clear from the foregoing investigation that NA abuse has found its way into the inner city. Poor, drug-involved, city dwellers are apparently not immune to the lure NAs have held for predominantly middle-class society. The evidence presented herein suggests that the appeal of NAs may exact a great price. Among other potential personal costs, drug overdose and a range of serious health and psychiatric conditions are associated with NA abuse in the inner city. The fact that the use of NAs is now commonplace among young and old alike reflects the alarming rise in the illicit use of NAs nationwide, and underscores the compelling need for further concentrated research into the incidence, prevalence and consequences of their use.

REFERENCES

Cone, E., Fant, R., Rohay, J., Caplan, Y., Ballina, M., Reder, R., Spyker, D. & Haddox, J. (2003). Oxycodone involvement in drug abuse deaths: A DAWN-Based classification scheme applied to an oxycodone postmortem database containing over 1000 cases. *Journal of Analytical Toxicology*, 27, 57-67.

Darke, S., Ross, D., Zador, D. & Sunjic, S. (2000). Heroin-related deaths in New South Wales, Australia, 1992-1996. *Drug and Alcohol Dependence*. 60, 141-150.

Drug Enforcement Administration Office of Diversion Control. *OxyContin diversion & abuse*. October, 2003.

Iguchi, M., Handelsman, L., Bickel, W. & Griffiths, R. (1993). Benzodiazepine and sedative use/abuse by methadone maintenance clients. *Drug and Alcohol Dependence*, 32, 257-266.

Janofsky, M. Drug-Fighters turn to rising tide of prescription abuse. *The New York Times*, March 18, 2004. *http://www.nytimes.com.*

Miller, N. & Greenfield, A. (2004). Patient characteristics and risk factors for development of dependence on hydrocodone and oxycodone. *American Journal of Therapeutics*, 11, 26-32.

National Institute on Drug Abuse. *Epidemiologic trends in drug abuse: Advance report*. Community Epidemiology Work Group, 6/2003.

Osam-O-Gram: Part I: Prescription analgesic abuse–Patterns of prescription analgesic abuse and perceived risks. Key findings from Ohio Substance Abuse Monitoring Network (OSAM) 6/2003 meeting. Available at *http://www.state.oh.us/ada/odada. htm.*

Osam-O-Gram: Part II: Prescription analgesic abuse–Initiation patterns and reported reasons for abuse. Key findings from Ohio Substance Abuse Monitoring Network (OSAM) 6/2003 meeting. Available at *http://www.state.oh.us/ada/odada.htm.*

Rooney, S., Kelly, G., Bamford, L., Sloan, D. & O'Connor, J. (1999). Co-abuse of opiates and benzodiazepines. *Irish Journal of Medical Science*, 168, 36-41.

Siegal, H., Carlson, R., Kenne, D. & Swora, M. (2003). Probable relationship between opioid abuse and heroin use. *American Family Physician.* Letter to editor, 3/1/2003.

Simoni-Wastila, L., Ritter, G. & Strickler, G. (2004). Gender and other factors associated with the nonmedical use of abusable prescription drugs. *Substance Use & Misuse* 39 (1), 1-23.

Simoni-Wastila, L. & Strickler, G. (2004). Risk factors associated with problem use of prescription drugs. *American Journal of Public Health,* 94 (2), 266-268.

Singer, M. & Weeks, M. (1996). Preventing AIDS in communities of color: Anthropology and social prevention. *Human Organization,* 55 (4): 488-492.

Substance Abuse and Mental Health Services Administration, Office of Applied Studies. *The DAWN Report: Narcotic analgesics,* January, 2003. Available at *http://www.DrugAbuseStatistics.samhsa.gov.*

Substance Abuse and Mental Health Services Administration, Office of Applied Studies. *The DASIS Report: Treatment admissions involving narcotic painkillers,* December 26, 2003. Available at *http://www.DrugAbuseStatistics.samhsa.gov.*

Substance Abuse and Mental Health Services Administration, Office of Applied Studies. *The national household survey on drug abuse (NHSDA) report: Nonmedical use of prescription-type drugs among youths and young adults,* January 16, 2003. Available at *http://www.DrugAbuseStatistics.samhsa.gov.*

Response to Trauma
in Haitian Youth at Risk

Richard Douyon, PhD
Louis Herns Marcelin, PhD
Michèle Jean-Gilles, PhD
J. Bryan Page, PhD

SUMMARY. In order to characterize undesirable behavior (drug use, fighting, criminal activity) among Haitian youth at risk and determine the relationship between traumatic experience and that kind of behavior, investigators recruited 292 Haitian youths via networks of informal social relations in two zones of Miami/Dade County strongly identified with Haitian ethnicity. Each recruit responded to an interview schedule eliciting sociodemographic information and self-reported activities, in-

Richard Douyon is affiliated with the University of Miami Department of Psychiatry and Behavioral Sciences.

Louis Herns Marcelin is affiliated with the University of Miami Department of Anthropology, and Department of Epidemiology and Public Health.

Michèle Jean-Gilles is affiliated with the Florida International University, College of Health and Urban Affairs.

J. Bryan Page is affiliated with the University of Miami Department of Psychiatry and Behavioral Sciences, Department of Anthropology, and Department of Sociology.

Address correspondence to: J. Bryan Page, University of Miami, Department of Anthropology, 102 Merrick (LC2005), Coral Gables, FL 33124 (E-mail: Bryan.page@miami.edu).

The authors wish to thank the National Institute on Drug Abuse for its support of this research through grant #1RO1 DA 12153.

[Haworth co-indexing entry note]: "Response to Trauma in Haitian Youth at Risk." Douyon, Richard et al. Co-published simultaneously in *Journal of Ethnicity in Substance Abuse* (The Haworth Press, Inc.) Vol. 4, No. 2, 2005, pp. 115-138; and: *New Drugs on the Street: Changing Inner City Patterns of Illicit Consumption* (ed: Merrill Singer) The Haworth Press, Inc., 2005, pp. 115-138. Single or multiple copies of this article are available for a fee from The Haworth Document Delivery Service [1-800-HAWORTH, 9:00 a.m. - 5:00 p.m. (EST). E-mail address: docdelivery@haworthpress.com].

Available online on http://www.haworthpress.com/web/JESA
doi:10.1300/J233v04n02_06

cluding involvement in youth-dominated groups. They also reported traumatic experience. Clinicians administered CAPS to a subset of those respondents who self-reported traumatic experience. Staff ethnographers selected respondents for in-depth interviews and family studies to provide contextual depth for findings of the interview schedule and the CAPS assessments. Although traumatic experience may still play a role in mental health outcomes among children, childhood victimization among Haitian children does not appear to be related to the drug use and undesirable behaviors associated with unsupervised youth, including formation of gangs. *[Article copies available for a fee from The Haworth Document Delivery Service: 1-800-HAWORTH. E-mail address: <docdelivery@ haworthpress.com> Website: <http://www.HaworthPress.com> © 2005 by The Haworth Press, Inc. All rights reserved.]*

KEYWORDS. Haitians, trauma, drug selling

INTRODUCTION AND BACKGROUND

Haitians in Miami have had the misfortune of encountering some of the most daunting barriers ever presented to an immigrant group. Not only have some of them made the trip to South Florida in the flimsiest of craft through dangerous seas, but many have sojourned for months or years under hostile conditions in the Bahamas before finally making their way to Miami. Once on shore in Dade County, the new arrivals have faced a community that has routinely ghettoized populations of color during most of its existence. Urbanized areas have well-defined zones inhabited by people of African descent whether they are North American, Bahamian, Jamaican, or other Caribbean. Although all housing is officially open by law, the population of the County clearly has compartmentalized phenotypes by geographic areas (Dunn, 1997; Peacock, Morrow, and Gladwin, 1997; Portes and Stepick, 1993). In this kind of racialized setting, the continued marginalization of a population descended from enslaved Africans hardly surprises.

Factors that have exacerbated this tendency to marginalize Haitian immigrants in Miami/Dade County include their supposed linkage with disease and superstition, and recently, association with juvenile crime. Just as the population of Haitian immigrants achieved a recognizable size and cohesion, about 1982, they registered on the Centers for Disease Control's monitors for the newly emergent disease complex, AIDS (Nachman and Dreyfus, 1986). Haitian immigrants' tuberculosis also brought them unwanted attention from North American health and im-migration authorities (Nachman, 1993). Some authors (e.g., Moore and LeBaron, 1986) hinted darkly that Haiti had been a major conduit for HIV into the United States. Later analyses of the pandemic have shown the reverse to be true (Farmer, 1998). Nevertheless, the early indication by the CDC that having Haitian background constituted a risk factor for AIDS did gratuitous and irreparable damage to the Haitian com-munity's image, especially in South Florida. This blaming of Haitians as unclean, disease-ridden interlopers has led to ongoing prejudice against them, and it has moved them, as a community, to distrust over-tures by researchers, especially if the researchers want to study AIDS or tuberculosis (Wingerd and Page, 1997).

Conditions of poverty, unemployment, and underemployment have persisted in South Florida's Haitian population despite the notable willingness of these newcomers to spend additional energy acquiring schooling that had not been available in Haiti. Although gathering large-scale demographic data on the Haitian population in South Florida presents difficulties (see Stepick and Stepick, 1990), it has become clear that a large proportion of that population still lives in conditions of over-crowding and poverty (Stepick and Stepick, 1992). The location of these Haitian Americans in the mix of ethnicities living in Dade County is contiguous with neighborhoods inhabited by other groups that had been marginalized earlier, including African Americans and African descended Caribbean people. This location is hostile territory, espe-cially for Haitian children trying to attend public schools in these neigh-borhoods. Furthermore, the lifeways of the "host" cultural context in which these children attempt to learn how to become "Americans" often communicate the futility of education and the attractiveness of "outlaw" or "gangsta" life, perhaps as a reflection of the "host's" own marginal-ity. Formation of youth gangs has occurred among almost every cultur-ally distinctive immigrant group that has arrived in the United States since 1860 (Goldstein, 1990), but under the conditions described above, the specific adaptations of inner city Haitian youth in the U.S. demand close examination.

The present study of Haitian Youth in Miami/Dade County attempts to define the responses of these youth to a hostile social and economic environment. Although the literature on gangs provides numerous tem-plates for characterizing these responses (cf. Arnold, 1965; Cloward and Ohlin, 1955; Cohen, 1960; Elliott, Ageton, and Canter, 1979; Fagan, 1989; Furfey, 1926; Goldstein, 1991; Thrasher, 1927), we shall attempt here to use self-reported and observed behaviors to define the adaptations of Haitian youth, holding in abeyance our comparisons of these adaptations with those in the rest of the literature.

Our preliminary work in preparing to study the emergent phenomenon of reported drug use and gang activity among Haitian youth first led us to examine the reports of these activities for veracity. Community contacts at the Center for Haitian Studies reported that some of the at-risk youth participating in their street diversion projects claimed to belong to gangs. Newspaper reports, beginning in 1996, described criminal activity among Haitian youth, a group that previously had not demonstrated much inclination toward delinquency of any kind. Conferences with gang specialists in the Metro-Dade County police force and the forces of local municipalities in Miami and North Miami Beach identified approximately 20 "gang entities" that had some of the characteristics of youth gangs seen in other parts of Miami/Dade County. These characteristics included having a recognizable name for the group, involvement in fighting, and criminal behavior involving drugs. Rather than accepting these descriptions as starting points for our investigation, we collected them for later comparison with our own experience with the intention of developing our own taxonomy of peer-dominated groups among Haitian youth. This taxonomy is still under development.

Previous work in the Haitian community revealed traumatic experience as a frequently reported feature of young Haitians' lives. In the course of other studies (Wingerd and Page, 1997), we found that some young Haitians had experienced notable trauma in a number of different contexts, including witness to political killings and torture, death of fellow travelers on the journey to the United States, mistreatment in holding camps and temporary quarters, and abuse at the hands of stepparents.

Because we realized that response to traumatic experience can reduce a person's ability to concentrate (Yehuda et al., 1995), which in turn would interfere with their performance in school, we theorized that Post-Traumatic Stress Disorder (PTSD) might help to explain heavy involvement in peer-dominated and drug-involved social groups (Duke et al., 2003). Our pilot assessments of a group of seven at-risk Haitian youths using the Clinician Administered Post-Traumatic Stress (CAPS) interview had the intention of detecting the presence of symptoms or diagnosability in this population (Blake et al., 1990). We found that all but one of the seven youths assessed by a child psychiatrist either had symptoms or were diagnosable with PTSD. We therefore proposed to broaden our study of PTSD among Haitian youth as a possible explanation for difficulties in school and delinquent behavior.

Brief Description of Gangs

In the course of intervening among Haitian youth for the prevention of HIV infection, a local community-based organization, the Center for Haitian Studies, began to receive reports from the participants in the intervention that Haitian young people had engaged in activities such as street-level drug trafficking, organized fights with other youths, and wearing of "colors." Some Haitian youths identify themselves as members of groups that use the word "zo" (Creole for "bone") in their names to express that they are "Haitian to the bone." These group names often take the forms: "Zo (location), or "Zo (address)," or "(attribute) Zo," or "(noun) Zo." In behavior and concept, the zo groups appeared to be gangs. News coverage of gangs in the community showed that what are now called Haitian gangs had not attracted any public attention before about 1994 (cf. Herald Staff, 1988, 1994, 1996, 1997).

Theory of Drug Involvement and Gang Development

When Haitians arrive in Miami, a place with a reputation of not being hospitable to people who are black and poor, they lack the proficiency in English and other educational characteristics to be eligible for any but the lowest-paying jobs. Too quickly, Haitian immigrants find themselves in the least desirable jobs, barely able to meet their family's basic needs with what they earn. In their encounters with the "native" population, they hear and see evidence that they are not held in high regard by their neighbors. This prejudice is linked to their skin color, but it extends to accusations of bringing disease. To add a final degree of difficulty to the process of adjustment, there are few extended family members available to moderate the stress and burden of immigrant status in daily life, no aunt Marie to take the children when one has to work late, no grandmother to spoil them, no community to monitor their behavior.

To varying degrees, the racial prejudice, lack of education, accusations of bringing disease, and lack of extended family resources affect all Haitian immigrants in South Florida, yet most have succeeded in making some sort of life without resorting to crime or delinquent activity. According to our theory, those who become involved in crime and delinquent behavior may have something more in their backgrounds, the experience of trauma.

The clinical construct most strongly identified with traumatic life experience is Post Traumatic Stress Disorder (Kessler et al., 1995) which holds that traumatic life events are processed on an unconscious level (for the "structural violence" variant of this theory, see Baer, Singer, and Susser, 2003: 213-216). When they have been too severe and/or persistent in the life of the individual, the memories of traumatic events can interfere with the functioning of adaptive mechanisms on cognitive, emotional, and behavioral levels (Brenner et al., 1995; Breslau et al., 1992; Yehuda et al., 1995).

Post-Traumatic Stress Disorder (PTSD) can be an extremely debilitating condition that occurs after exposure to a terrifying event or ordeal in which grave physical harm occurred or was threatened. Traumatic events that can trigger PTSD include violent personal assaults such as rape or mugging, natural or human-caused disasters, accident, or military combat. Survivors of traumas, people who witnessed traumatic events, and families of victims are among those who develop PTSD (Romero-Daza and Singer, 1997; Romero-Daza, Weeks, and Singer, 2003).

Many people with PTSD repeatedly reexperience the ordeal in the form of flashback episodes, memories, nightmares, or frightening thoughts, especially when they are exposed to events or objects reminiscent of the trauma. Anniversaries of events can trigger symptoms. People with PTSD also experience emotional numbness and sleep disturbances, depression, anxiety, and irritability or outbursts of anger. Feelings of intense guilt are also common. Most people with PTSD try to avoid any reminders or thoughts of the ordeal. PTSD is diagnosed when symptoms last more than one month.

About 3.6% of U.S. adults (5.2 million people) have PTSD during the course of a given year (NIMH, 2004). PTSD can develop at any age, including in childhood. Symptoms typically begin within three months of a traumatic event, although occasionally they do not begin until years later. Once PTSD occurs, the severity and duration of illness vary. Some people recover within six months, while others suffer much longer. Co-occurring depression, alcohol or other drug abuse, or another anxiety disorder are not uncommon. The likelihood of treatment success is increased when these conditions are appropriately diagnosed and treated. People who have been abused as children or who have had other previous traumatic experiences are more likely to develop the disorder.

Nevertheless, not all people who have traumatic experiences develop symptoms of PTSD. Cultural background and social support (cf. Eisenman et al., 2003), history of head trauma (Keenan et al., 2003), and hippocampal volume (Gilbertson et al., 2003) may affect whether or not people exposed to trauma develop symptoms. Experience with trauma may be more likely in some cultural contexts than in others. For example, people living in Israel or some parts of the developing world have high rates of exposure to violent acts (Eisenman et al., 2003). How people respond to traumatic experience may vary from one cultural context to another. Israelis exposed to terrorism demonstrated rates of PTSD symptoms similar to those found in Guatemalans 20 years after traumatic experience (Bleich, Gelpoff, and Solomon, 2003; Sabin et al., 2003). Detection of traumatic experience and diagnosis of PTSD may present added difficulties in culturally distinct populations (Eisenman et al., 2003).

We theorized that young people who have seen terrible acts of violence or gruesome events, or who live in the thrall of abuse in their own homes would exhibit some symptoms linked with PTSD that would predict poor performance in school, anti-social behavior, and violence. Intrusive thoughts about trauma would disrupt attention in school, either directly, or indirectly through sleep disturbance. Attempts to use drugs to prevent or moderate these symptoms could ensue. Startle reactions and defensive behavior would attract attention and ridicule of fellow students. This array of difficulties, coupled with feeling embattled in surroundings populated by people of different cultural backgrounds might result in the youth's seeking social contexts in which participants have similar life experiences and are similarly angry and frustrated about them. Individuals with these characteristics could easily be expected to form peer-controlled groups that engage in delinquent behavior, or, as they are often called, gangs. Recent research on moderation of the effects of trauma on children (cf. Stein et al., 2003) indicates that if the preceding ethologic theory were correct, cognitive behavioral intervention might have the effect of preventing this kind of behavior. The study described here attempted to focus attention on traumatic experience among Haitian youth as a strategy for understanding the emerging formation of peer-controlled groups that engaged in drug-selling and other delinquent activity.

METHODS

Participants

We spent three years identifying and recruiting 292 Haitian youths at risk through direct, street-based contact with networks of informal social relations. Each of the new recruits, after a consent procedure involving parents of those under 18 years of age, responded to an interview schedule consisting of questions on sociodemographic characteristics, immigration history, self-reported involvement in use of illegal drugs, involvement in peer-dominated social groups, and traumatic life experiences. The latter set of questions inquired about the participants' exposure to parental abuse, forcible sex, witnessing death or serious injury by accidental or intentional violence, serious illness, or imprisonment. If the respondents answered in the affirmative to any of these questions, they became eligible for a later administration of the CAPS.

Because the interview schedule's sensor for traumatic experience tended to include rather than exclude, we could reasonably expect a significant portion of the included respondents not to show symptoms for PTSD. The 228 people identified as having experience with trauma included 29% who only had one variety of trauma to report, but this criterion for identifying traumatic experience did not reflect duration, intensity, or severity of that experience. A person exposed to constant beatings and threat of physical harm over two years had different reasons for showing signs of Post-Traumatic Stress Disorder than a person who had witnessed a single violent incident, yet both would show the same number of traumatic experiences in our crude sensor. The CAPS provided an opportunity to characterize traumatic experience in terms of variety, frequency, or intensity. Although it would have been ideal to administer the CAPS to all individuals who self-reported traumatic experience in their responses to the interview schedule, we were able to do so only with a subset of these individuals.

Several problems in re-recruitment of this subpopulation presented barriers to their continued participation, including change of address before the field team could recontact them, difficulties in scheduling the administration of the CAPS, and refusal to participate in the second stage of the study. A total of 47 of the 228 participants who had a history of traumatic experience took part in the CAPS.

Procedures and Assessment of Trauma

The Clinical Assessment of PTSD Severity (CAPS) is a structured interview that has demonstrated reliability for detecting symptoms of PTSD and measuring its severity (Blake et al., 1990). The Structured Clinical Interview for DSM-IV (SCID) (First et al., 1996) is the standard method for reliably diagnosing PTSD and ruling out other Axis I disorders. The investigators used it to rule out anxiety disorders other than PTSD, mood disorders, psychosis, and drug-use disorders. The Bellevue Adolescent Interview schedule (BAIS) (Lewis et al., 1988) assesses child abuse in both physical and sexual victimization. It distinguishes between physical and sexual abuse and helps to compare the impact of these two types of trauma. A psychiatrist, with the help of one other clinician, administered these instruments to a total of 47 study participants. The clinicians administering the CAPS received training in its administration at the same time from the same instructor, Dr. Daniela David of the University of Miami's Department of Psychiatry and Behavioral Sciences. This training included establishment of high reliability among raters through repeated practice administrations.

Analyses

Responses to the structured interview were entered into an SPSS file for analysis, producing frequency distributions of sociodemographic characteristics of the study population. The item-by-item responses to the CAPS as well as summary scores also were entered into an SPSS file and that was merged with the structured interview file for the purpose of comparing CAPS respondents with non-respondents. Summary CAPS scores were hypothesized to be independent variables predicting self-reported gang involvement, as well as violent and delinquent behavior.

RESULTS

The team of field workers recruited 291 respondents from whom they gathered sociodemographic and self-reported data on risk and delinquent behavior to contextualize the clinical assessments performed by the clinicians. Table 1 shows that the participants included 35% females, and the participants' ages ranged from 12 to 25, with 70%19 or under. Two-thirds of the participants in the structured interview were teenage boys born in the U.S., and 91.7% of the participants, when asked about their primary cultural identification, identified themselves as Haitians or Haitian-Americans. The remaining 8% had claimed some form of Haitian identity during the recruitment process, but when responding to the formal question they identified African American, Black, Bahamian, or "other." Preliminary work had identified three terms to identify groupings of Haitian youths not supervised by adults: gang, clique, and group. More than one-third of the participants had taken part in activities of one or more of these agglomera-

TABLE 1. Age and Sex of Participants

| | | SEX | | Count | |
		MALE	FEMALE	Total	%
Age at	12	1	1	2	0.7
Interview	13-14	9	10	19	6.5
	15-17	42	58	100	34.4
	18-22	113	32	145	49.8
	23-up	22	3	25	8.6
Total		187	104	291	100.0

tions, and 15% were currently active in a self-identified gang at the time of the interview. Most of them were exposed to gangs, cliques or groups and their activities early in their teenage years, between 12 and 15 years old, specifically during middle school.

Youths recruited from Homestead/Florida City were significantly more likely to report traumatic experience than those recruited in Little Haiti (see Table 2). Accidents and natural disasters were by far the most frequently reported traumatic experiences for the total group reporting trauma (Table 3). Among the individuals assessed for PTSD (see Table 4), assault by strangers was the most frequently reported source of trauma, but it was not strongly associated with PTSD symptoms or other psychological problems.

Assault by family members and assault by police were two varieties of trauma reported by the respondents to the CAPS (see Table 5). Respondents who reported these kinds of assaults attributed great distress to them. Of the CAPS respondents, 71% received a total CAPS score of one or higher (range of CAPS–frequency 1-55; combined frequency and intensity 2-109; intensity 1-57). Of these individuals, 13 were diagnosable and one more was symptomatic but not diagnosable for PTSD. Symptoms reported by these individuals (both diagnosed and symptomatic) included memory lapses, outbursts of anger, and emotional distress.

The relationships among traumatic experience, traumatic disorder, and delinquent behavior did not emerge from the data as theorized. Self-reported gang affiliation and experience with trauma were not re-

TABLE 2. Trauma by Neighborhood

Count

		NEIGHBORHOOD			
		LITTLE HAITI	HOMESTEAD	Total	%
TRAUMA	NO	52	11	63	21.6
	YES	149	79	228	78.4
Total		201	90	291	100.0

Chi-square = 6.827 P = .009

TABLE 3. Self-Reports of Trauma

Types of Trauma	N*	%
War Zone	6/228	2.6
Sex with Older Person	52/228	22.8
Imprisonment	45/228	19.7
Serious Accident	115/228	50.4
Natural Disaster	171/228	75.0
Life Threatening Illness	37/228	16.2
Sexual Assault by Family Member	8/228	3.5
Assault by Family Member	39/228	17.1
Sexual Assault by Stranger	25/228	11.0
Assault by Stranger	59/228	25.8
Forced into Sex	27/228	11.8
Forced into Sex by You	8/228	3.5

*Respondents reported more than one variety of trauma, so numerators add up to more than 228.

lated (Chi-square = 1.811, P = .404), nor was self-reported drug use related to traumatic experience (Chi-square = .135, P = .713; see Table 6). Similarly, experience with trauma was not related to specific delinquent activities, such as carjacking, burglary, drug dealing, or robbery, using dichotomous versions of the summary traumatic experience variable and the delinquent behavior variables. In the 47 cases where the participants' traumatic experiences were more thoroughly characterized by

TABLE 4. CAPS and SCID Results

Trauma	N*	%
War Zone	4/47	8.5
Sex with Older Person	14/47	29.8
Imprisonment	31/47	66.0
Torture	6/47	12.8
Serious Accident	16/47	33.3
Natural Disaster	27/47	55.6
Life Threatening Illness	11/47	23.4
Sexual Assault by Family Member	6/47	12.8
Assault by Family Member	15/47	31.9
Sexual Assault by Stranger	4/47	8.5
Assault by Stranger	32/47	68.9

*Respondents reported more than one variety of trauma, so numerators add up to more than 47.

TABLE 5. Traumas Causing the Most Distress

Triggering Traumas	N*	%
War Zone	1/47	2.1
Imprisonment	4/47	8.5
Torture	1/47	2.1
Serious Accident	4/47	8.5
Natural Disaster	1/47	2.1
Life Threatening Illness	1/47	2.1
Sexual Assault by Family Member	3/47	12.8
Assault by Family Member	9/47	19.1
Sexual Assault by Stranger	1/47	2.1
Assault by Stranger	7/47	14.9
Other Traumatic	11/47	23.4
Did not find any of these experiences distressing	4/47	8.5

TABLE 6. Relationships (Chi-square) Between Traumatic Experience and Delinquent Behavior

Self-reported Behavior	Yes	No	Chi-square	Significance
Former affiliation with gang	95	192*	1.595	P = .450
Current affiliation with gang	45	243*	1.811	P = .404
Current affiliation with clique	33	217**	2.820	P = .420
Current affiliation with group	8	242**	2.563	P = .464
Does current gang/ clique fight?	56	20***	.332	P = .255
Have you fired a gun in a fight?	32	70***	1.249	P = .264
Gang/clique dealt drugs in last 12 mo.	58	52***	3.006	P = .222
Gang/clique carjack in last 12 mo.	47	64***	2.019	P = .364
Gang/clique burglary in last 12 mo.	38	73***	1.517	P = .468
Gang/clique robbery in last 12 mo.	41	70	1.597	P = .450

TABLE 6 (continued)

Self-reported Behavior	Yes	No	Chi-square	Significance
Gang/clique used mj in last 12 mo.	80	33***	4.625	P = .201
Gang/clique used Coc. in last 12 mo.	11	102***	2.644	P = .450
Gang/clique used Heroin in last 12 mo.	2	111***	2.488	P = .477
Gang/clique used Crack in last 12 mo.	7	106***	2.164	P = .539
Respondent ever dealt drugs	62	225	4.174	P = .124
Respondent ever car-jacked	26	260	6.844	P = .033[a]
Respondent ever burglarized	28	258	2.865	P = .239
Respondent ever robbed	31	255	3.120	P = .210
Respondent ever used illegal drugs	113	174	.135	P = .713
Respondent ever used Marijuana	110	174	.850	P = .654
Respondent ever used Cocaine	18	269	2.649	P = .266
Respondent ever used Crack	2	285	.643	P = .725

[a] Respondents without traumatic experience were significantly more likely to have personally participated.
*Total does not equal 292 because of refusals to answer.
**Total does not equal 292 because not all youths recognize all terms for youth groups.
***Analysis included only respondents with current or historic affiliation with gangs, cliques, or groups.

the CAPS score and diagnostic criteria, the relationships between the effects of trauma and specific aspects of delinquent behavior also proved not to be statistically significant (see Table 7).

Slightly fewer than one-third of the CAPS interviewees, all of whom had traumatic experience, met criteria for PTSD, and one additional individual was assessed to have some symptoms of that disorder (see Table 8). More than one-quarter of the CAPS respondents (13) had zero scores on the CAPS, demonstrating no apparent effects of their self-reported traumatic experiences that included seeing a brother drown, having a friend who was shot to death, being hit by a car, and being flooded out by Hurricane Andrew. The trauma of individuals with zero scores on the CAPS involved natural disasters, attacks by police or other strangers, or sex with a person more than five years older than the respondent. Nevertheless, some individuals with scores on the CAPS had single traumatic experiences of short duration.

In an attempt to probe the intensity of delinquent behavior among CAPS respondents, the investigators constructed a composite score of that behavior by combining self-reports of seven different varieties of delinquent behavior, including fighting, carjacking, auto theft, robbery, drug trafficking, burglary, and fencing of stolen goods. This composite score was also statistically unrelated to CAPS score ($R = .275$, R-square = 0.076; $F = 2.045$, Sig. = 0.165), or diagnosis of PTSD ($F = 1.359$, Sig. = 0.255).

We pursued the alternative hypothesis that a specific aspect of the symptoms attributed to PTSD might predict violent behavior among youths with traumatic experience. A separate part of the CAPS involves irritability and sudden violence, and we used this variable to attempt to predict the array of undesirable behaviors presented earlier. Table 9 presents the individual behaviors studied in this analysis, which produced no significant relationships. We also analyzed the composite variable of combined self-reported behaviors, and the one-way ANOVA yielded an F of .726. Regardless of how we constructed bivariate analyses, among the Haitian youth recruited into this study, we could find no relationship between delinquent behavior and PTSD and its symptoms.

How these youth came to circumstances in which they were exposed to abuse by household members and brutal treatment by police appears to depend primarily on how they and their families have fared after immigration, rather than what happened before or during that process. The following clinical notes taken during the administration of the Clinician-administered post-traumatic stress (CAPS) illustrate the participants' perceptions of their traumatic experiences.

TABLE 7. Relationships (ANOVA) Between CAPS Score and Delinquent Behavior

Self-reported Behavior	Yes	No	F	Significance
Former affiliation with gang	18	28*	.266	P = .609
Current affiliation with gang	16	30*	.828	P = .424
Current affiliation with clique	6	26**	.703	P = .501
Current affiliation with group	2	30**	1.228	P = .303
Does current gang/ clique fight?	15	5***	.206	P = .815
Have you fired a gun in a fight?	11	15***	.533	P = .473
Gang/clique dealt drugs in last 12 mo.	19	9***	.387	P = .682
Gang/clique carjack in last 12 mo.	15	13***	.575	P = .567
Gang/clique burglary in last 12 mo.	13	15***	1.659	P = .202
Gang/clique robbery in last 12 mo.	16	12***	1.085	P = .347

TABLE 7 (continued)

Self-reported Behavior	Yes	No	F	Significance
Gang/clique used mj in last 12 mo.	24	6***	.270	P = .765
Gang/clique used Coc. in last 12 mo.	5	25***	.353	P = .704
Gang/clique used Heroin in last 12 mo.	1	29***	.624	P = .541
Gang/clique used Crack in last 12 mo.	2	28***	.604	P = .521
Respondent ever dealt drugs	18	29	.748	P = .392
Respondent ever car-jacked	9	38	.294	P = .590
Respondent ever burglarized	9	38	.011	P = .918
Respondent ever robbed	10	37	1.525	P = .223
Respondent ever used illegal drugs	26	20	1.219	P = .275
Respondent ever used Marijuana	26	20	1.219	P = .275
Respondent ever used Cocaine	6	40	1.010	P = .373
Respondent ever used Heroin	1	45	1.267	P = .292
Respondent ever used Crack	2	44	1.058	P = .356

*Total does not equal 47 because of refusals to answer.
**Total does not equal 47 because not all youths recognize all terms for youth groups.
***Analysis included only respondents with current or historic affiliation with gangs, cliques, or groups.

TABLE 8. CAPS Results

	Yes	%	No	%	Symptoms/ Sub-threshold	%	Total
Diagnosis of PTSD	13	27.6	33	70.2	1	2.1	47
Self-Report of Memory Lapses	6	12.8	35	74.5	6	12.8	47
Self-Report of Angry Outbursts	12	25.5	31	66.0	4	8.5	47
Self-Report of Emotional Distress	11	23.4	26	55.3	10	21.2	47

TABLE 9. Relationship Between Outbursts of Anger and Violent Behaviors

	Yes	No	Total	Chi-square	P
Gang membership	15	28	43	1.601	.659
Car jacking	8	35	43	0.839	.840
Burglary	8	35	43	3.675	.299
Auto theft	14	29	43	4.114	.249
Robbery	10	33	43	2.198	.532
Fired gun in fight	11	31	42	0.342	.559

Case #1

A 16-year-old boy witnessed his 1-year-old sister raped by a family friend two years ago. The friend was never caught. He felt used by the friend. He carries feelings of guilt.

Case #2

The boy says that being stabbed was an act of injustice because police did not do anything about it even though he told them where to find the person at school. His attacker was never arrested. He also said, if it were he [who had been accused] he would have been arrested; he still wants revenge.

Case #3

At age 1, this female teenager was forced into sex with the next door neighbor while the aunt was working. The neighbor was a friend and trusted by the aunt to watch over her. Also, her uncle once walked into the bathroom while she was taking a shower and talked to her about sex. She became terrified of the uncle.

Case #4

He saw his little brother pushed into the lake and drowned in front of him. He was pushed into the water, too, but was saved after swallowing a lot of water. He feels lucky to be alive. He has guilty feelings and anger about this incident.

Case #5

This 20-year-old male witnessed a "lady friend" getting shot in front of him. The police never showed up, even after they called several times. Referring to the police, he said, "It's all about the system. The system is set up a way to mess everything up. It's all Babylon. This society is about only the strong who can survive. It's not about black and white anymore."

Case #6

This boy was hit in the head by his father and sustained a long gash. The father is in jail now. The boy feels responsible. He saw his father hit in the head by someone else a year ago.

Case #7

While resisting arrest, this boy had sustained a broken leg at age 9. He also sustained a broken arm and a skull fracture by his mother at age 11 and 12 respectively. He was involved in shoplifting and car theft at an early age.

These clinician's assessments take the violent incidents in the study participants' backgrounds out of context, pointing out their key features and alluding to an aftermath. Responses of the young people in these seven cases vary, from guilt in cases 6 and 1, to cynicism in case 5, to desire for revenge in case 2, to ongoing terror in case 3. All responses hold the potential for future harm to the victim. The guilty feelings expressed by the boy in case 6, on the most immediate level may cause him to feel that he deserves further physical abuse, if he remains in the living arrangement in which his father injured him. In both cases 6 and 1, the youths' guilt may lead to feelings of reduced self-worth, which can in turn lead to self-destructive behavior and even suicide. The cynicism shown in case 5 is apparently channeled into a broader condemnation of "Babylon" in Rastafarian style. The boy who wants revenge may resort to violence, and the young woman who is afraid of men and sex may have major problems in adapting to adult life. These residual feelings, however, do not necessarily translate into measurable disorder, and even measurable disorder does not predict delinquent behavior.

DISCUSSION

The administration of the CAPS to people from a cultural background as distinctive as that of Haitians would seem to present problems of language and cultural interpretation, but in fact, the young Haitians encountered in street environments primarily spoke English. None were monolingual Creole speakers. Furthermore, the pretest revealed no difficulties in administering the CAPS to young, English-speaking Haitians. In the absence of full translation, back-translation, and item-by-item checks for cultural appropriateness, we cannot assume that the administration of the CAPS was completely without misunderstandings of a cultural nature. Nevertheless, the data presented here suggest that no systematic problems with administrations occurred during this study. Responses varied significantly, and the summary scores ranged from 0 to 109 with scores distributed throughout the range, suggesting wide variation in frequency and intensity of response to traumatic experience.

The lack of any demonstrable relationship between CAPS scores or PTSD diagnosis and involvement in delinquent behavior or unsupervised groupings of Haitian youth suggest that the process of entering and sustaining this kind of activity has a much subtler relationship with traumatic experience than we originally hypothesized. At minimum, we can conclude that traumatic experience as measured by CAPS is neither a necessary nor sufficient cause of joining gang-like groups or engaging in delinquent activity. Just because the CAPS and SCID instruments do not detect the effects of trauma, however, does not mean that trauma has not had some other kind of impact on those who have experienced it. Recent studies by DeBelles (2002), Heim and Nemeroff (2001), and Yehuda (2001) suggest that, especially in children, traumatic experience causes the nervous system to assume a state of constant arousal that is not susceptible to measurement by means of accepted methods. This subtle, sub-clinical state may be related to misuse of drugs (DeBelles, 2002) or anxiety disorders (Heim and Nemeroff, 2001). We cannot assume that the Haitian youths who have had a traumatic experience now live with a state of constant arousal, but such a state could help to explain the receptivity of some youths to the overtures of their delinquent peers. In the absence of a measurement for detecting this subtle condition, we can only speculate on its effects based on correlations with misuse of drugs (cf. DeBelles, 2002) and anxiety (cf. Heim and Nemeroff 2001).

Findings of very recent studies in populations heavily exposed to trauma but variable in PTSD and its symptoms (Bleich, Gelpoff, and Solomon, 2003; Sabin et al., 2003; Stein et al., 2003) suggest that people from culturally distinct groups may have ways of handling traumatic experience that affect the rates at which PTSD is detectable among them. Our results would place Haitian youth between the Latin Americans and the Israelis in this gradient of response to traumatic experience.

On the other hand, the two-thirds of study participants who took part in the CAPS assessment did not meet criteria for PTSD. Furthermore, the clinicians' qualitative assessments of their conduct in the interviews found most of them to have normal social skills and no outward signs of psychopathology. Most responded to uncomfortable questions with grace and calm, and they presented themselves as having adapted to their difficult situations. This information gives rise to another hypothesis about the emergence of gang-like and delinquent behavior among these young people–that they represent attempts by human beings who are not yet mature to adapt to difficult circumstances of socioeconomic status, truncated extended family, race/ethnic stigma, and traumatized history, among other serious problems. The present study has collected data on these environmental factors, and will address them in subsequent articles.

CONCLUSIONS

Although traumatic experience may still play a role in mental health outcomes among children, childhood victimization among Haitian children does not lead inevitably to PTSD, and it does not appear to be related to the undesirable behaviors associated with unsupervised youth, including formation of gangs. Youngsters who demonstrate high resilience to the effect of serious trauma require further study to differentiate among reaction to trauma that is not measurable by existing instrumentation, intrapsychic resilience, and culturally patterned resilience. A prospective study to assess responses of Haitian youth to stressors found in their local immigrant communities would help to identify appropriate interventions that address these stressors and moderate responses to them. Response to trauma may have more importance in Haitian youth than CAPS-detectable PTSD, necessitating detection of low cortisol, and high CRF and norepinephrine levels in response to stress and trauma. The present study engaged in none of these assessments, but they could be important in unraveling the relationship between trauma and undesirable behavior among Haitian youth.

REFERENCES

Arnold, W. R. (1965) The concept of gang. *Sociological Quarterly* 7 (1), 59-75.

Blake, D. D., Walther, F. W., Nagy, L. M., Kaloupek, D. G., Klauminzer, G., Charney, D. S. & Keane, T. M. (1990) A clinician rating scale for assessing current and lifetime PTSD. *Behavior Therapist,* 13, 168-188.

Bleich, A., Gelpoff, M. & Solomon, Z. (2003) Exposure to terrorism, stress related mental health symptoms, and coping behaviors among a nationally representative sample in Israel. *JAMA* 290 (5), 612-620.

Brenner, J. D., Randall, P., Scott, T. M., Bronen, R. A. et al. (1995) MRI-based measurement of hippocampal volume in patients with combat-related posttraumatic stress disorder. *American Journal of Psychiatry* 152 (7), 973-981.

Breslau, N., Davis, G. C., Andreski, P. & Peterson, E. (1992) Traumatic events and posttraumatic stress disorder in an urban population of young adults. *Archives of General Psychiatry* 48: 216-222.

Cloward, R. A. & Ohlin, L. E. (1960) *Delinquency and opportunity: A theory of delinquent gangs.* New York: Free Press.

Cohen, A. K. (1955) *Delinquent boys: The culture of the gang.* New York: Free Press.

DeBelles, M. D. (2002) Developmental traumatology: A contributory mechanism for alcohol and substance use disorders. *Psychoneuroendocrinology* 27: 155-170.

Duke, M., Teng, W., Simmons, J. & Singer, M. (2003) Structural and interpersonal violence among Puerto Rican drug users. *Practicing Anthropology* 25 (3): 28-31.

Dunn, M. (1997) *Black Miami in the twentieth century.* Gainesville: University of Florida Press.

Eisenman, D. P., Gelberg, L., Liu, H. & Shapiro, M. F. (2003) Mental health and health related quality of life among adult Latino primary care patients living in the United States with previous exposure to political violence. *JAMA*, 290, no. 5, 627-634.

Elliott, D. S., Ageton, S. S., & Canter, R. J. (1979) An integrated theoretical perspective on juvenile delinquency. *Journal of Research in Crime and Delinquency.* 16, 3-27.

Fagan, J. (1989) The social organization of drug use and drug dealing among urban gangs. *Criminology* 27 (4), 633-667.

Farmer, P. (1998) *Infections and inequalities.* Berkeley: University of California Press.

First, M. B., Gibbon, M., Spitzer, R. L. & Williams, J. B. (2002) *Instruction manual for the Structured Clinical Interview for DSM-IV.* New York: New York State Psychiatric Institute.

Furfey, P. H. (1926) *The gang age.* New York: Macmillan.

Goldstein, A. P. (1989) *Delinquent gangs: A psychological perspective.* Champaign, IL: Research Press.

Heim, C. & Nemeroff, C. (2001) The role of childhood trauma in the neurobiology of mood and anxiety disorders: Preclinical and clinical studies. *Biological Psychiatry.* 49, 1023-1039.

Herald Staff (1988) Nature of gangs in Dade County. *Miami Herald,* September 18.

_____ (1994) Marginalization and despair: Haitian youths in Little Haiti. *Miami Herald,* June 12.

_____ (1996) Gang warfare stokes fear in Little Haiti. *Miami Herald,* 1st part, August 10, 2nd, August 18.

_____ (1997) Taped beating a gang ritual? Neighbor films teenagers' fighting in Miramar. *Miami Herald,* December 18.

Keenan, H. T., Runyan, D. K., Marshall, S. W., Nocera, M. A., Merten, D. F. & Sinai, S. H. A. (2003) Population-based study of inflicted traumatic brain injury in young children. *JAMA,* 290, no. 5, 621-626.

Kessler, R. C., Sonnega, A., Bromet, E., Hughes, M. & Nelson, C. B. (1995) Posttraumatic Stress Disorder in the national comorbidity survey. *Archives of General Psychiatry* 52, 1048-1060.

Lewis, D. O., Pincus, J. H., Bard, B. et al. (1988) Neuropsychiatric, psychoeducational, and family characteristics of 14 juveniles condemned to death in the United States. *American Journal of Psychiatry* 145, 584-589.

Marcelin, L. H. & Marcelin, L. M. (n. d.) Childhood and the definition of the domestic domain. Unpublished manuscript.

Moore, A. & LeBaron, R. (1986) The case for a Haitian origin of the AIDS epidemic. In D. Feldman & T. Johnson (eds.) *The Social dimensions of AIDS: Method and theory*, pp. 77-93. New York: Praeger.

Nachman, S. (1993) Wasted lives: Tuberculosis and other health risks of being Haitian in a US detention camp. *Medical Anthropology Quarterly* 7, 227-259.

Nachman, S. & Dreyfus, G. (1986) Haitians and AIDS in South Florida. *Medical Anthropology Quarterly* 17, 32-33.

NIMH (2004) Post-traumatic Stress Disorder–Web Page: http://www.nimh.nih.gov/publicat/reliving.cfm.

Page, J. B. (1997) Vulcans and Jutes: Cuban fraternities and their disappearance. *Free Inquiry in Creative Sociology* 25 (1): 65-74.

Peacock, W., Morrow, B. & Gladwin, H. (1997) *Hurricane Andrew: Ethnicity, gender and the sociology of disaster*. London: Routledge.

Portes, A. & Stepick, A. (1993) *City on the edge: The transformation of Miami*. Berkeley: University of California Press.

Romero-Daza, N. & Singer, M. (1997) Another type of victim: Witnessing violence and drug initiation among Puerto Ricans in Hartford. Paper presented at the annual meetings of the American Anthropological Association, Washington, DC 1997.

Romero-Daza, N., Weeks, M. & Singer, M. (2003) "Nobody gives a damn if I live or die." Experiences of violence among drug-using sex workers in Hartford, CT. *Medical Anthropology* 22 (3): 233-259.

Sabin, M., Lopes Cardoso, B., Nackerud, L., Kaiser, R. & Varese, L. (2003) Factors associated with poor mental health among Guatemalan refugees living in Mexico 20 years after civil conflict. *JAMA* 290 (5), 635-642.

Stein, B. D., Jaycocks, L. H., Kataoka, S. H., Wong, M., Tu, W., Elliott, M. N. & Fink, A. (2003) A mental health intervention for school children exposed to violence. *JAMA* 290 (5), 603-611.

Stepick A. (1992) The refugees nobody wants: Haitians in Miami. In G.J. Grenier & A. Stepick (eds.) *Miami now!* pp. 57-82. Gainesville, FL: University Press of Florida.

Stepick, A. & Stepick, C. (1990) People in the shadows: Survey research among Haitians in Miami. *Human Organization* 49 (1), 64-77.

Thrasher, F. (1927) *The gang*. Chicago: University of Chicago Press.

Wingerd, J., & Page, J. B. (1997) HIV counseling for Haitian women: Culturally sensitive approaches. *Health Education & Behavior* 24 (6), 736-745.

Yehuda, R. (2001) Biology of Posttraumatic Stress Disorder. *Journal of Clinical Psychiatry* 62 [suppl 17], 41-46.

Yehuda, R., Keefe, R. S. E., Harvey, P. D., Levengood, R. A., Geber, D. K., Geni, J. & Siever, L. J. (1995) Learning and memory in combat veterans with posttraumatic stress disorder. *American Journal of Psychiatry* 152 (1): 137-139.

Index